Clinical Testing of the Vestibular System

Advances in Oto-Rhino-Laryngology

Vol. 42

Series Editor
C.R. Pfaltz, Basel

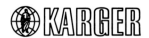

Basel · München · Paris · London · New York · New Delhi · Singapore · Tokyo · Sydney

Selected Papers of the Bárány Sociey Meeting, Bologna,
June 1–4, 1987

Clinical Testing of the Vestibular System

Volume Editor
E. Pirodda, Bologna

118 figures, 1 color plate and 37 tables, 1988

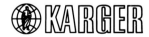

Basel · München · Paris · London · New York · New Delhi · Singapore · Tokyo · Sydney

Advances in Oto-Rhino-Laryngology

Library of Congress Cataloging-in-Publication Data
Bárány Society. Meeting (1987: Bologna, Italy)
Clinical testing of th vestibular system.
(Advances in oto-rhino-laryngology; vol. 42)
Includes bibliographies and index.
1. Vestibular Apparatus-Congresses. 2. Vesti-
bular Apparatus-Diseases-Diagnosis-Congresses.
3. Vestibular Function Tests-Congresses.
I. Pirodda, Ettore. II. Title. III. Series.
[DNLM: 1. Vestibular Apparatus-Physiology-
Congresses. 2. Vestibular Function Tests-
Congresses. W1 AD701 v. 42 / WV 255 B225c 1987]
RF16.A38 vol. 42 617'.51 s 88-13048
[RF260] [617.8'82]
ISBN 3-8055-4767-6

Bibliographic Indices
This publication is listed in bibliographic services, including Current Contents® and Index Medicus.

Clinical Testing of the Vestibular System

This volume contains 61 selected papers presented at the Bárány Society Meeting, Bologna, June 1–4, 1987. 44 further papers are published as "Neurophysiology of the Vestibular System", forming vol. 41 in the series Advances in Oto-Rhino-Laryngology (for contents see pp. IX–XI).

Contents

Contents VI

Neurophysiology of the Vestibular System

44 selected papers presented at the Bárány Society Meeting, Bologna, June 1–4, 1987. Published as vol. 41 in the series Advances in Oto-Rhino-Laryngology.

Contents

Contents

Adv. Oto-Rhino-Laryng., vol. 42, pp. 1–4 (Karger, Basel 1988)

Vestibulo-Ocular Reflex and Optokinetic Nystagmus in Microgravity

Gilles Clément, Alain Berthoz[1]

Laboratoire de Physiologie Neurosensorielle du CNRS, Paris, France

Evidence that sustained linear accelerations can modify nystagmus elicited by stimulation of the semicircular canals has been reviewed by Benson [1974]. There is also evidence that sinusoidal linear acceleration can modulate velocity of nystagmus slow phases elicited by a constant velocity optokinetic stimulus [Buizza et al., 1980]. However, all these observations are limited because of the difficulty of applying a simple linear acceleration on Earth where the gravitational field is present and introduces a permanent bias. Microgravity induced by orbital or parabolic flight is an elegant way to suppress the gravity vector selectively. We have therefore used this condition to study its influence, and consequently the otolithic contribution to the vestibulo-ocular reflex (VOR) and the optokinetic nystagmus (OKN).

VOR elicited by active head oscillation was tested daily on one subject throughout a space mission of the US Space Shuttle Discovery in June 1985. The results showed a strong decrease of both horizontal and vertical VOR gain in darkness at the beginning of the flight [Viéville et al., 1986]. The drop of gain observed during pitch head motion in microgravity would reveal the contribution of the otoliths to the vertical VOR. Another possibility is that astronauts would not be able to imagine a Shuttle-fixed target during head oscillation in darkness because of the absence of an effective static gravitational vector. It was also proposed that the subject actively suppressed VOR because of an intralabyrinthine conflict resulting from the difficulty to interpret the otolith signal. Such suppression has also been observed on the first day of Spacelab-D1 mission: two astronauts performed an adequate compensatory horizontal eye movement during head oscillations but the

[1] The authors are grateful to M.F. Reschke and S. Wood (SBRI, NASA JSC, Houston) for their help with KC-135 inflight data collection.

slow phase gain was very low and the VOR was replaced by compensatory saccades [Von Baumgarten et al., 1986].

During the same space flight, OKN elicited by a monocular visual stimulator attached to the subject's head was measured daily in one astronaut, and on flight days 2, 4 and 7 in another. The major changes in the microgravity environment were the beating field and the gain of the OKN in the vertical plane [Clément et al., 1986]. At the beginning of the flight the beating field shifted progressively downward. Within 1 h after landing, there was a large drift of the beating field upward followed by large resets downward. Results also showed a reversal of the asymmetry of the vertical OKN gain at the beginning of the space flight: downward (slow phase up) OKN gain which was higher in normal gravity was lower in microgravity relative to upward (slow phase down) OKN gain. Casual measurements of optokinetic after-nystagmus (OKAN) showed an increase in time constant of downward (slow phase up) OKAN on the first in-flight day and from flight days 4 to 7.

These results clearly showed an effect of gravity on the asymmetry of vertical OKN gain. Such changes in the nystagmus slow phase component, observed in vertical and horizontal planes, might also be the result of a mechanism in the vestibular nuclei that stores integrated spatial orientation sensory information, including input from the visual and vestibular systems. However, these results have been obtained during orbital flight on 2 subjects only, and they needed further confirmation with other subjects.

In the present work, we have repeated this experiment during parabolic flight aboard NASA's KC-135 aircraft, yielding alternate two-g periods and zero-g periods, each lasting about 25 s. OKN was produced by a checkerboard pattern moving at constant velocity in front of the subject's right eye. The remarkable finding during parabolic flight is that when the visual pattern is moving either upward or downward, there is a downward drift of the beating field of the OKN (fig. 1). Indeed, during transition from two-g to zero-g the OKN is clearly superimposed on a large downward gaze deviation. This observation is consistent with the results of orbital flight on the downward drift of the beating field during the early exposure to microgravity. Also comparable with orbital flight data are the measurements of horizontal and vertical OKN gain obtained during zero-g periods with several subjects, showing a significant reversal of asymmetry of vertical OKN gain (fig. 2).

Our data are actually in contrast with those expected from ground experiments. Indeed, the results of Igarashi et al. [1978] who observed a slight increase in slow phase velocity in both upward and downward direc-

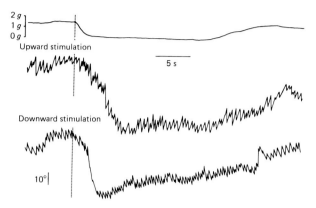

Fig. 1. Samples of vertical eye movements in response to upward and downward moving pattern recorded during parabolic flight. The signal recorded by an accelerometer placed along the body longitudinal axis (z-axis) is shown on the top trace.

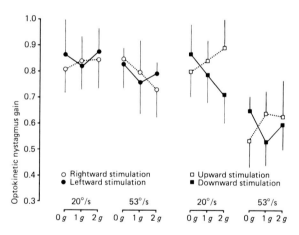

Fig. 2. Comparison between measurements of the OKN gain (mean values and standard deviation from 6 subjects) elicited by horizontal and vertical visual stimulation at constant velocity (20 and 53°/s) in normal gravity condition (1 g), and during zero-g and two-g phases of parabolic flight.

tions after saccular ablation in the monkey clearly suggest an inhibitory action of sacculus on OKN. Matsuo and Cohen [1984] also showed that the gain and time constant of downward (slow phase up) OKAN is increased during lateral head tilt and suggested that the gain and time constant of downward OKN should be increased when the gravity is reduced. One possible explanation of our findings would be that in normal gravity the sacculus exerts a general activation of all extensor muscles of neck and limbs. It would also tend to elevate the eye by an action on the extra-ocular muscles (superior rectus and inferior oblique), thus exerting an inhibitory action on downward eye movements. In microgravity, this upward drive would be suppressed and the eye would therefore tend to move downward. This would explain the downward gaze deviation and the enhancement of the velocity of the slow phases when directed downward.

References

Benson, A.J.: Modification of the response to angular acceleration by linear acceleration. Handbook of sensory physiology, vol. VI, 2, pp. 281–320 (Springer, Berlin 1974).

Buizza, A.; Léger, A.; Droulez, J.; Berthoz, A.; Schmid, R.: Influence of otolithic stimulation by horizontal linear acceleration on optokinetic nystagmus and visual motion perception. Exp. Brain Res. 39: 165–176 (1980).

Clément, G.; Viéville, T.; Lestienne, F.; Berthoz, A.: Modifications of gain asymmetry and beating field of vertical optokinetic nystagmus in microgravity. Neurosci. Lett. 63: 271–274 (1986).

Igarashi, M.; Takahashi, M.; Kubo, T.; Levy, J.K.; Homick, J.L.: Effect of macular ablation on vertical optokinetic nystagmus in the squirrel monkey. ORL 40: 312–318 (1978).

Matsuo, V.; Cohen, B.: Vertical optokinetic nystagmus and vestibular nystagmus in the monkey. Up-down asymmetry and effects of gravity. Exp. Brain Res. 176: 159–164 (1984).

Viéville, T.; Clément, G.; Lestienne, F.; Berthoz, A.: Adaptive modification of the optokinetic and vestibulo-ocular refexes in microgravity, in Keller, Zee, Adaptive processes in visual and oculomotor systems, pp. 111–120 (Pergamon Press, Oxford 1986).

Von Baumgarten, R., et al.: European experiments on the vestibular system during the Spacelab D-1 mission; in Sahm, Jansen, Keller, Scientific results of the German Spacelab Mission D1, pp. 477–490 (WPF c/o DFVLR, Köln 1986).

Gilles Clément, PhD, Laboratoire de Physiologie Neurosensorielle du CNRS, 15 rue de l'Ecole de Médecine, F-75270 Paris Cedex 06 (France)

Adv. Oto-Rhino-Laryng., vol. 42, pp. 5–8 (Karger, Basel 1988)

Spaceflight Affects the 1-g Postrotatory Vestibulo-Ocular Reflex[1]

Charles M. Oman, Mark J. Kulbaski[2]

Man Vehicle Laboratory, Massachusetts Institute of Technology, Cambridge, Mass., USA

Horizontal vestibulo-ocular reflex (VOR) changes were studied in 4 crew members (male, aged 35–53) of the 10-day space shuttle Spacelab 1 mission (November, 1983). Evidence that linear acceleration and head tilt can modify nystagmus elicited by angular stimulation [reviewed by Benson, 1974] is well known. Tilting the head results in a more rapid decay of after-nystagmus. Experiments conducted in brief 5- to 20-second parabolic flights have demonstrated no short-term changes in VOR gain in 0-g [Jackson and Sears, 1966; Vesterhauge et al., 1984]. However, results obtained by Lackner and Graybiel [1981] and by DiZio et al. [1987] are consistent with the view that the apparent long time constant of the VOR is shortened in weightlessness. The major questions addressed in the present study were: Does a prolonged exposure to weightlessness produce a residual alteration in the dynamics of the postrotatory VOR, as measured on the ground during the first several days postflight? Is it adaptive? Does prolonged weightlessness alter the effects of head tilt on the postflight VOR in 1-g?

VOR test sessions were conducted 151, 120, 65, 43, and 10 days preflight, and 1, 2, and 4 days postflight. Eye movements were recorded via bitemporal EOG on FM tape and later digitized for computer analysis. Subjects were blindfolded eyes open, and instructed to 'look straight ahead'. Alertness was continually maintained with conversation. In each session, the subject was rotated CW about a vertical axis for 1 min at 120°/s, stopped, and postrotational VOR was recorded for 1 min. This procedure was then repeated 3 times, alternating rotation directions. In the first two tests, the

[1] Supported by NASA Contract NAS9–15343.

[2] We thank Drs. L. Young, B. Cohen, A. Natapoff and K. Johnson, J. Gidney, E. Riskin, M. Massoumia, R. Renshaw, S. Modestino and our subjects.

subject maintained the head erect position throughout. In tests 3 and 4 ('dumping tests'), he pitched his head forward approximately 90° 5 s after chair stop, maintained this position for 5 s, and then resumed the head upright position. Nystagmus slow phase velocity (SPV) was calculated, and interpolated across fast phase intervals using an interactive computerized technique [Massoumnia, 1983]. Twenty-one of 145 records, and the first second of each run were discarded for technical reasons. Postrotatory data from the 5 preflight sessions, postflight days 1 and 2, and postflight day 4 were each averaged and compared, both for the group of 4 and for the individual subjects. Head erect SPV data was fit with a first-order model: response gain and apparent time constant (TC) were determined via log linear regression of average SPV versus time (1–20 s at 0.25-second intervals). A head pitched TC was calculated using a similar method on dumping test data between 5 and 10 s. Significance of differences between mean SPV profiles was assessed separately, using a χ^2 test, by calculating the ratio of squared difference in mean SPV to pooled variance at each point in time, and summing. The χ^2 significance test thus did not depend on the first-order model approximation we used to characterize our data.

For head erect postrotatory VOR, group SPV gain remained 0.59 both preflight and postflight. This value corresponds closely to that recently reported by Benson and Viéville [1986], who independently studied VOR gain in 2 of our 4 subjects before and after the same mission, and who gave the subjects similar gaze instructions. Average preflight and postflight head erect postrotatory responses are shown in figure 1 for our study. Preflight group TC was 12.8 s (range by subject: 7.4–16.7 s). However, 1–2 days postflight, the TC had shortened to 9.5 s (range: 4.9–13.9 s). TC shortening was seen in 3 of the 4 individual subjects. The increased rate of SPV decay was particularly prominent 6–20 s after chair stop, as shown in figure 1. A χ^2 test comparing the difference in the mean preflight and postflight group responses relative to their inherent variance indicated a significant ($p < 0.005$) difference during this epoch, whereas the first 1–5 s of data were indistinguishable. Four days postflight, the group TC had recovered to 12.3 s. We believe these changes are residual adaptive effects resulting from extended exposure to 0-g. Qualitatively similar changes in TC were recently described by DiZio et al. [1987] during (but not after) acute exposure to 0-g in parabolic flight. Because the changes persist for several days postflight, we tentatively attribute the changes seen to functional alterations in the CNS VOR velocity storage mechanism [Cohen et al., 1977] and not to inherent gravity sensitivity in semicircular canal responses. The hypothesized velocity

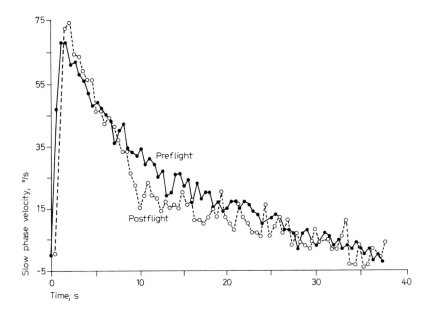

Fig. 1. Comparison of preflight and postflight (days 1, 2) head erect postrotatory VOR slow phase velocity, interpolated across fast phases and averaged across all subjects and trials.

storage mechanism is believed largely responsible for determining the SPV decay rate during the 6- to 20-second epoch, to be labile, and to be functionally dependent on vestibular, visual, and haptic sensory inputs. In the preflight dumping tests, the group TC (as measured between 5 and 10 s) was 3.6 s (range by subject: 3.1–8.7 s). Steepening of the TC upon head tilt in 1-*g* is consistent with previous results, and may be due to dumping of central velocity storage by vestibular or other inputs. Postflight, the head forward TC was 3.8 s (range: 1.3–4.8 s), indicating that the dumping phenomenon remained, despite 10 days exposure to an agravic environment.

References

Benson, A.: Modification of the response to angular accelerations by linear accelerations; in Kornhuber, Handbook of sensory physiology, vol. 6, part 2, pp. 281–320 (Springer, Berlin 1974).

Benson, A.; Viéville, T.: European vestibular experiments on the Spacelab-1 mission. 6. Yaw axis vestibulo-ocular reflex. Exp. Brain Res. *64:* 279–283 (1986).

Cohen, B.; Matsuo, V.; Raphan, T.: Quantitative analysis of the velocity characteristics of optokinetic nystagmus and optokinetic after-nystagmus. J. Physiol. *270:* 321 (1977).

DiZio, P.; Lackner, J.; Evanoff, J.: The influence of gravitoinertial force level on oculomotor and perceptual responses to sudden stop stimulation. Aviat. Space Envir. Med. *58:* suppl. A (1987).

Jackson, M.; Sears, C.: The effect of weightlessness upon the normal nystagmus reaction. Aerospace Med. *37:* 719–721 (1966).

Lackner, J.; Graybiel, A.: Variations in gravitoinertial force level affect the gain of the vestibulo-ocular reflex: implications for the etiology of space motion sickness. Aviat. Space Envir. Med. *53:* 154–158 (1981).

Massoumenia, M.-A.: Detection of fast phase of nystagmus using digital filtering; SM Thesis, Cambrige (1983).

Vesterhauge, S.; Mansson, A.; Johansen, T.S.: Vestibular and oculomotor function during Gz variations. Motion sickness: mechanisms, prediction, prevention, and treatment. CP-372:24, 1–4 (NATO/AGARD, Neuilly sur Seine 1984).

Charles M. Oman, PhD, Man Vehicle Laboratory, Massachusetts Institute of Technology, Rm 37–219, Cambridge, MA 01239 (USA)

Adv. Oto-Rhino-Laryng., vol. 42, pp. 9–12 (Karger, Basel 1988)

Pupil Size and Microgravity

W.J. Oosterveld[a], H.A.A. de Jong[a], J. Smit[b], H.W. Kortschot[b]

[a]University of Amsterdam, Amsterdam;
[b]National Aerospace-Medical Center, Soesterberg, The Netherlands

The eye possesses a dual motor innervation and its effects, induced by vestibular stimulation upon ocular reflexes, are always mixed because of impulses being conducted both through somatic and autonomic pathways. The motor control of the dilator pupillae is maintained by impulses from the posterior and lateral regions of the hypothalamus through the brain stem and cervical cord and back up through the cervical sympathetic chain, the ciliospinal ganglion of Budge [5].

The constriction of the pupil is a parasympathetic action through fibers originating in Edinger-Westphal's nucleus in the mesencephalon; the proganglionary fibers are part of the oculomotor nerve. The force of the constrictory muscles seems to be stronger than that of the dilatory muscles. The pupil size is influenced by many factors: accommodation, emotion, fatigue, eye movements, intraocular pressure, sleep, light supply as well as stimulation of other sensory organs as hearing and smell.

Semmlow et al. [11] found variations in pupillary responsiveness with pupil size as a nonlinear process. Selective utricular stimulation revealed that pupillary action showed a rhythmic pattern of dilatations and constrictions during and immediately after a period of nystagmus [4]. In order to investigate the effect of otolithic stimulation on pupillary size the eyes of human test subjects were investigated during parabolic flight.

Methods

The subjects were strapped into a chair, while their head rested on a pad in a small container where the illumination was sustained at a low intensity. At a distance of 60 cm the subjects had to stare at a light point. Before each experimental trial a rest period of at least 3 min was maintained. Continuous pupil observations of one eye were made with a

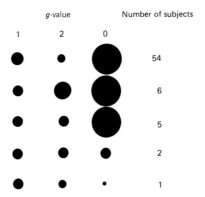

Fig. 1. Effect of *g*-value and weightlessness on pupil size.

video camera. All test subjects (68) were experienced with parabolic flight. The parabolas were flown with a Fokker F27. The periods of microgravity lasted approximately 10 s. Each person was subjected to at least 12 parabolas, with 20 recordings per parabola.

The effect of microgravity and the increased *g*-load prior to and following the parabolas was not similar in all subjects. A dilatation meant an increase in diameter of more than 10%, a constriction a decrease of more than 10%.

Results

In 65 out of a total of 68 subjects microgravity gave a dilatation of the pupil (fig. 1). Of the 3 other cases in 2 there was no reaction at all and in one a constriction. An increase of the *g*-load resulted in a constriction in 55 cases, a dilatation in 6 cases and no effect in 7 cases. The onset of pupillary action occurred with the introduction of zero-*g*. However, as the onset of the microgravity differed between the parabolas, no reliable data about this aspect could be collected. In 3 subjects the pupil size was measured during an exposure to a *g*-load up to 2.8 *g* in a human centrifuge at the Soesterberg Aerospace-Medical Centre. All subjects showed a constriction, followed by a dilatation when the accelerative force was lowered to the 1-*g* condition again.

Discussion

Emotional and sensory stimulations are able to provoke a dilatation of the pupil [10, 13]. In the present study the emotional factors were excluded as the subjects were experienced. Vestibular afferents are linked to the intraocular muscles via one or both sets of autonomic fibers derived from the superior cervical or ciliary ganglion [1]. The cervical trunk of the sympathetic nerve receives strong impulses after vestibular stimulation [2, 12].

The reflex regulation of pupillary size is attributed more to fluctuations in the discharge through the ciliary ganglion than to sympathetic innervation. The dilatation and constriction of the pupil is due to alterations in parasympathetic activity [6, 7]. Morrison and Pompeiano [8] found that the medial and descending vestibular nuclei play a role in pupillary dilatation.

DeSantis and Gernandt [3] stimulated the utricles both in cats and squirrel monkeys, resulting in brisk conjugate deviations of the eyes, accompanied by pupillary reactions. The fast phase of the eye movements went together with a pupillary constriction, the slow phase with a dilatation. Changes both in pupillary size and heart rate are completely abolished following vestibular lesions [8, 9].

The effect of microgravity and increased g-load on pupillary size is hard to explain. Besides the direct utricular fibers to the Edinger-Westphal area, more synaptic connections are probably due to the phenomenon. Nearly every reflex mechanism has a purpose. However, the purpose of the described reflex phenomenon is not clear at all.

References

1 Christensen, K.: Sympathetic and parasympathetic nerves in the orbit of cat, J. Anat. 70: 225–232 (1936).
2 Cobbold, A.F.; Megighian, D.; Sherrey, J.H.: Vestibular evoked activity in autonomic motor outflows. Arch. ital. Biol. 106: 113–123 (1968).
3 DeSantis, M.; Gernandt, B.E.: Effect of vestibular stimulation on pupillary size. Expl Neurol. 30: 66–77 (1971)
4 Gernandt, B.E.: Nystagmus evoked by utricular stimulation. Expl Neurol. 27: 90–100 (1970).
5 Kalyanaraman, S.: Some observations during stimulation of the human hypothalamus. Confinia neurol. 37: 189–192 (1975).
6 Lowenstein, O.; Loewenfeld, I.E.: Role of the sympathic and parasympathic systems in reflex dilatation of the pupil. AMA Archs Neurol. Psychiat. 64: 313–340 (1950).
7 Lowenstein, O.; Loewenfeld, I.E.: Mutual role of sympathic and parasympathic in shapening of the pupillary reflex to light. AMA Archs Neurol. Psychiat. 64: 341–377 (1950).
8 Morrison, A.R.; Pompeiano, O.: Vestibular influences on vegetative functions during the rapid eye movement periods of desynchronized sleep. Experienta 21: 667–668 (1965).

9 Morrison, A.R.; Pompeiano, O.: Vestibular influences during sleep. VI. Vestibular control of autonomic functions during the rapid eye movements of desynchronized sleep. Arch. ital. Biol. *108:* 154–180 (1970).
10 Rumpf, G.: Pupillary reaction while smelling and hearing. Proc. Congr. Orbital Diseases, Amsterdam 1973.
11 Semmlow, J.; Hansmann, D.; Stark, L.: Variation in pupillomotor responsiveness with mean pupil size. Vision Res. *15:* 85–90 (1975).
12 Tang, P.C.; Gernandt, B.E.: Autonomic responses to vestibular stimulation. Expl Neurol. *24:* 558–578 (1969).
13 Walsh, F.B.; Hoyt, W.F.: Clinical neuro-ophthalmology; 3rd ed., vol. 1, p. 482 (Williams & Wilkins, Baltimore 1969).

W.J. Oosterveld, MD, University of Amsterdam, Academisch Medisch Centrum, Meibergdreef 9, NL-1105 AZ Amsterdam (The Netherlands)

Adv. Oto-Rhino-Laryng., vol. 42., pp. 13–17 (Karger, Basel 1988)

Pre- and Postflight (D-1) Postural Control in Tilting Environments

W. Bles[a,b], J.L. van Raay[a]

[a]TNO Institute for Perception, Soesterberg; [b]Department of Otolaryngology, Free University Hospital, Amsterdam, The Netherlands

The goal of this study was the pre- and postflight assessment of the weighting of the otolith information by studying the influence of tilting visual surroundings on spatial orientation and on upright stance.

The principle of the tilting room is as follows: The subject is standing in the middle of the room on a fixated horizontal platform. Since the room tilts laterally from the base, the visual information is exactly the same whether the subject or the room is tilting laterally. So room tilt suggests body tilt into the opposite direction which might lead to a visually induced body correction in the direction of the room tilt. However, since the gravity vector is not changed the otolith information is at odds with the visual information: there is no need for a vestibularly induced body correction. Recording of the resulting body sway may reveal the weighting of the visual and otolith information in postural control: a large body sway indicates dominance of vision, a small sway dominance of the otolith system. Such a set-up proved to be useful in monitoring compensation processes after labyrinthine lesions [Bles et al., 1983] and also in the case of motion sickness susceptibility [Bles et al., 1985]. For this reason the test has been included in the pre- and postflight data acquisition programme of the D1-mission incorporated in the set of experiments (coded ES201) by the consortium of European investigators (P.I.: R.J. von Baumgarten, University of Mainz). From previous space flights we know that postflight postural balance could be impaired [Young et al., 1985]. The goal of this experiment was to record the time course back to normal postural stabilization together with the weighting of the information of the different sensory systems.

Apparatus and Procedure

The tilting room is a completely closed device (2.5 × 2.5 × 2 m) except for the entrance in the front wall and a part of the floor. In the middle of the floor is a hole which contains a force-measuring platform in fixed horizontal position for measurement of the anterior-posterior and left-right body sway of the subjects. The room is tilted sinusoidally with an amplitude of 5° and frequencies of 0.025, 0.05, and 0.2 Hz. Just before the back wall of the room a bar is positioned which tilts around the rotation axis of the room with an amplitude of 1.5° at a fixed frequency of 0.05 Hz. The subject is instructed to stand upright and to align the bar with the gravity vector by means of a potentiometer he holds in his hand. The tilt of the room and the bar is computer-controlled as is the data acquisition.

The whole procedure, including the reference measurements in a stable visual surround and in darkness, i.e. with eyes closed, took about 15 min per subject. Since the measurements were repeated with the subjects standing on top of a layer of foam rubber in order to enhance the effects, the total measurement time per subject took maximally 30 min.

Preflight measurements took place at Köln (at L-120 and L-86) and at Kennedy Space Center (at L-46 and L-18). The postflight measurements at KSC were performed on day R+1, R+2 and R+5. On day R+0 2 of the science astronauts (PS2 and PS3) were examined at Dryden in a simplified tilting room. The main difference was that there was no bar to keep in a vertical position.

Results

The effect of room tilt on the subjective vertical has been analyzed by computing the Fourier component of the bar settings at the stimulus frequencies. An ANOVA showed a mean amplitude of 3.1° re true vertical for 4 of the astronauts (quite considerable in view of the 5° room tilt) and one significantly smaller amplitude of 1.5° for PS3. No effect was found between the pre- and postflight settings and no effect of using foam rubber. Finally, only a frequency effect was found, showing smaller amplitudes with 0.2 Hz, which is understandable because of the difficulties in adjusting the bar at these fast room movements.

The effect of room tilt on postural control was examined by computing the Fourier component of the left-right stabilogram at the stimulus frequency. Except for the measurement on day R+0, the induced postural sway was very small for all astronauts. They were all below the 5th percentile of the normal control population. Figure 1 shows the original stabilometric recordings and the respective Fourier spectra of PS2 and PS3 at day L-18, R+0 and R+1 for the stimulus frequency of 0.2 Hz. PS3 had problems in the tilting

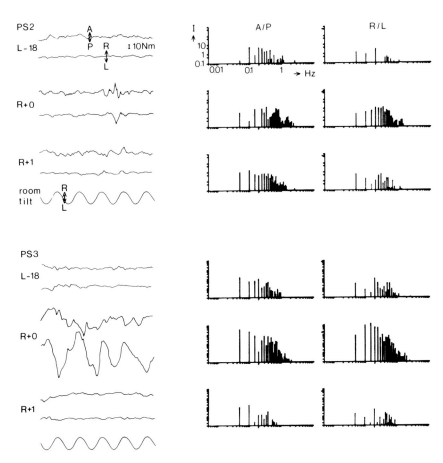

Fig. 1. Original stabilometric recordings and Fourier power spectra obtained in the tilting room at 0.2 Hz from PS2 and PS3 at days L-18, R+0 and R+1.

room at day R+0 and even lost his balance at this frequency, most probably because he perceived the room as stationary, but on day R+1 he was extremely stable. PS2 showed a different behavior: he could resist the room tilt be it at the cost of considerable muscle effort, visible in the left-right as well as in the fore-aft stabilogram (high frequency components). This is still visible on day R+1 and even on day R+5 (not shown) in the fore-aft sway. PS2 and PS3 showed the same behavior when standing on foam rubber although more enhanced.

The analysis of the recordings on foam rubber revealed a training effect especially with the lower frequencies which were interrupted only on day R+0 and to some extent on day R+1 with 2 of the 5 astronauts.

Closing the eyes in the reference measurements on day R+0 did not disturb postural balance in such a way that balance could not be maintained, even when standing on foam rubber. The resulting disturbance in the stabilogram after eye closure, however, did not reveal a strategy typical for all astronauts.

Conclusions

(1) The results of the dynamic rod-and-frame test (i.e. the adjustment of the bar in the tilting room) were postflight not different from preflight, suggesting that the otolithic-visual interaction in the perception of the vertical is back to normal within one day after a flight of 8 days.

(2) On day R+0 different weighting of the sensory information was observed in the tilting room for PS2 and PS3. PS3 seems to be more visually oriented than PS2 in view of the finding that PS3 did not observe room tilt on day R+0, in line with the results of other D-1 experiments [Friederici and Levelt, 1986].

(3) Postflight postural instability was not as bad as expected. For the 2 astronauts considered, 5 h postflight balance could be maintained while standing on foam rubber with the eyes closed. This is at odds with previous reports from astronauts about an immediate falling over after eye closure.

(4) Return to preflight behavior in the tilting room was extremely fast. It looks as if the astronauts, because of their rich vestibular history, have learnt to selectively pick up the appropriate available sensory information. The observed postural instability in the tilting room on day R+0 is most probably indeed an aftereffect of the previous microgravity conditions of the vestibular system since the tilting room has no effect on trained subjects after 10' days absolute bed rest, neither in the low nor in the high frequency region.

Acknowledgements

The authors acknowledge the programmatic support provided by the Netherlands Agency for Aerospace Programs and the Sled Experimenter Team at Mainz and, last but not least, the cooperation of the D1-astronauts Dunbar, Bluford, Messerschmid, Furrer, Ockels and Merbold.

References

Bles, W.; Jong, H.A.A. de; Oosterveld, W.J.: Prediction of seasickness susceptibility. AGARD Conf. Proc. No. 372, 27: 1–6 (1985).

Bles, W.; Vianney de Jong, J.M.B.; Wit, G. de: Compensation for labyrinthine defects examined by use of a tilting room. Acta oto-lar. *95:* 576–579 (1983).

Friederici, A.D.; Levelt, W.J.M.: Cognitive processes of spatial coordinate assignment. Naturwissenschaften *73:* 455–458 (1986).

Young, L.R.; Watt, D.G.D.; Oman, C.M.; Money, K.F.; Lichtenberg, B.K.: Spatial orientation in weightlessness and readaptation to earth's gravity. AGARD Conf. Proc. No. 377, 2: 1–6 (1985).

W. Bles, MD, TNO Institute for Perception, PO Box 23, NL-3769 ZG Soesterberg (The Netherlands)

Adv. Oto-Rhino-Laryng., vol. 42, pp. 18–23 (Karger, Basel 1988)

Determinants of Space Perception in Space Flight

Horst Mittelstaedt

Max-Planck-Institut für Verhaltensphysiologie, Seewiesen, FRG

This contribution deals with the event, well documented in space flight, that an astronaut experiences himself *and* the familiar room oriented upside down, even though he floats upright relative to the room, that is, even though his Z-axis is in alignment with the normally vertical polar axis of the room. I suggest to name an inversion phenomenon like this, that is, an inversion, which occurs in spite of or in the absence of external cues for the vertical, a 'cue-free inversion' (CFI). The question is, what may be its cause?

(1) At normal gravity, only those of our mechanoreceptors can tell us whether we are upright or upside down, which are sensitive to the Z-component of the gravity vector, that is, the component parallel to our, normally vertical, long axis. Now assume, for the sake of argument, that the CNS is able to compute, from the output of all gravity receptors, three variables which are each exclusively dependent on one of the three orthogonal components of the force-vector. When the X- and Y-vector components are zero, in the upright position, the state of the X- and Y-variables will then indicate the vertical, and very precisely, as testified by the precision with which a healthy person can keep balance. These two are unable to discriminate between the upright and the inverted posture, however, because they are then in the same state. It is exactly that state in which they are also at zero-*g*. Which of the two positions is then finally indicated must therefore depend on what is signalled by the Z-variable when the Z-force component is zero.

(2) This can be determined at normal gravity by placing the subjects on the tiltable board of figure 1 and asking them to change by remote control the angle of roll tilt ρ, in total darkness, until they feel to be completely horizontal. The subject is fitted with a personal bite board, which is oriented at 90° to the board in the two positions of the subject, right ear down or left ear down, respectively. The means of these two series of mesurements are

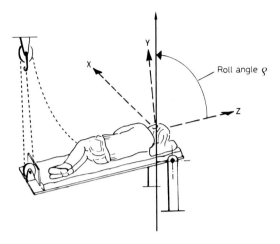

Fig. 1. Set-up for measuring the subjective horizontal position. The subject, head fixed by means of bite-board (not visible in figure), may rotate the board about X-axis by remote control until she/he feels to be in a horizontal position.

averaged as $\check{\rho}=\frac{1}{2}(\bar\rho r \text{-} \bar\rho e)$ [for details, see Mittelstaedt, 1987]. A healthy subject is able to indicate her/his subjective horizontal position $\check{\rho}$ (SHP) with an SD of $0.8 \pm 0.2°$ and with a deviation from $\check{\rho}=90°$, which is usually significant though rarely more than $5°$, and stays fairly constant for a given subject over many years.

Consider a person who feels to be horizontal, if, as in figure 1, she lies tilted at $\check{\rho}<90°$. When such a subject is placed into an objectively horizontal position, that is, when the Z-axis-force component is zero, the Z-variable must now indicate a *head-down* posture. Exactly this message must result at zero-*g*, then, and consequently, the CNS cannot but decide the open alternative 'upright or upside down' in favour of the latter. The opposite decision must ensue for a subject who evinces an SHP of $\check{\rho}>90°$.

The signal which causes the deviation of the SHP from $\check{\rho}=90°$ must be rather small compared to the maximal static Z-axis response at normal gravity. Its quantity, relative to the latter, is measured as the negative cosine of $\check{\rho}$. Its absolute mean is only $4.2 \pm 3.3\%$ (n=44 subjects). Yet, at zero-*g*, it is the only gravity variable which differs from its null position, and hence the only one that may decide the polarity of the vertical. Physiologically, it is very likely due to an imbalance of the resting discharges of the Z-axis receptors. It shall be called 'postural bias'. Available space does not permit to go into the details of the theory here, which are (see p. 24 this volume

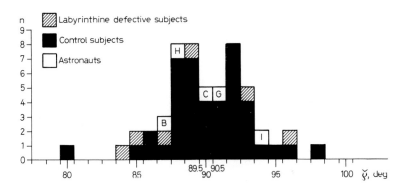

Fig. 2. SHP (p̆, in degrees) of 44 control subjects, 6 labyrinthine-defective subjects, and 5 astronauts, labelled by code letters as in figure 3 and table I.

[Mittelstaedt and Fricke, 1988]) complicated by the differential roles of saccules and somatoreceptors, as well as by the effect on the subjective vertical of the 'idiotropic vector'. The effect of the latter, fortunately, is in all subjects tested not large enough (M<0.6) to reverse the effect of a negative saccular bias at zero-*g*, though it will weaken the stability of the decision.

(3) It is to be expected therefore that the postural bias and hence the SHP is negatively correlated with the occurrence of a CFI. Figure 2 shows the SHP of 5 astronauts of the two spacelab missions (coded in compliance with US Privacy Act), as part of an SHP histogram of control subjects. Except in subject C, all deviations from p̆=90° are highly (p<0.005; two-tailed) significant. Subjects B and H, who evince a negative bias, have both reported a CFI, B directly after orbit insertion, H after he had left his sleeping bunk on his first 'morning'. Subject C has repeatedly testified his inability to experience any direction as vertical; 'up' and 'down' had lost any phenomenal reality for him. Subject I, by contrast, has stated emphatically that 'up' was always in the direction of his head, such that, when he floated inclined relative to the spacelab, the spacelab looked tilted whereas he felt upright. Subject G did not report a CFI at orbit insertion or after getting up in the morning, but later on experienced varying reference directions. Therefore, the statistics are computed also without G's data and without accounting for C's indifference. Table I shows correlation coefficients r between SHP and CFI as well as the probability p that r is only by chance at least that much different from zero *and* negative. Despite the small sample the correlations have reached (or at least approached) significance.

Table I. Comparison of SHP and postural bias with occurrence of cue-free inversion (CFI): correlations r and probabilities p (see text) are compute evaluating C's indifference as zero (ternary rating) or as minus 1 (binary rating), respectively, as well as including or excluding G data

1	Subjects ranked according to line 2		B	H	C	G	I		correlation with p̂ (line 2)	
									r	p
2	SHP p̂, °		86.9	88.3	89.8	91.3	93.5			
3	Postural bias, % of max		−5.4	−3.0	−0.4	+2.3	+6.1			
					not significant					
4	CFI		yes	yes	no	no	no		no	no
					indifferent					
		ternary								
		all	+1	+1	0	−1	−1		−0.933	0.01
		without G	+1	+1	0	−	−1		−0.971	0.014
5	CFI rating	binary								
		all	+1	+1	−1	−1	−1		−0.837	0.039
		without G	+1	+1	−1	−	−1		−0.823	0.088

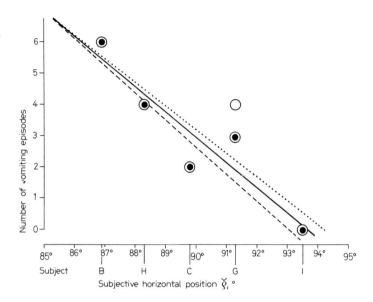

Fig. 3. Number of vomiting episodes as a function of SHP (p̆). Regressions are computed also inclusive of provoked episode (○; dotted line), and excluding G data (dashed line).

The CFI did not recur to B and H later on in the flight. But even at the end of the mission, their spatial perception differed characteristically from that of the 3 others. The latter (notably subject I) had no difficulties when they floated inverted relative to spacelab, to see the objective ceiling as 'subjective floor' in a perceptual switch of the Necker cube type (called 'visual reorientation episode' by Oman et al. [1986]). By contrast, B and H could confessedly never do that trick to their satisfaction.

Clearly, then, subjects with a negative postural bias are more often confronted with conflicting orientational cues than their counterparts. Since sensory conflict is thought to be among the causes of earthbound motion sickness, I have checked whether, in these 5 subjects, there is a negative correlation between postural bias and symptoms of space sickness. And this is in fact true for a number of indicators of the malaise. A crude but rather well-defined indicator is the number of vomiting episodes. In figure 3, it is plotted as a function of the SHP. Subject G has tried to intentionally elicit a vomiting episode on his second day. Independently of whether this provoked (fourth) episode is included or not, the correlation, and hence the regression, is significant with p=0.012–0.034. Also, expectedly, there is a clear-cut *positive* correlation between the number of vomiting episodes and CFI.

(4) The present results are compatible with the hypothesis that a resting discharge bias of the Z-axis receptors determines the SHP and the CFI. How the bias may influence the probability of occurrence and the intensity of space malaise symptoms is an open question. The CFI, at any rate, even though likely to enhance the malaise, is neither necessary nor sufficient to release it. But there may be another causal link: in weightlessness, a negative postural bias is bound to severely disturb the transformation of head-fixed information into trunk-fixed coordinates, and head roll or pitch is well known to be provocative.

Regardless of their causes the correlations, if found reliable, open new opportunities for space medicine, e.g. for the selection of astronauts who have to be top fit from the start. Also, the compensation of a postural bias by means of a spatial training might be feasible.

References

Mittelstaedt, H.: Inflight and postflight results on the causation of inversion illusions and space sickness; inSahm, Jansen, Keller, Proc. Norderney Symp. on Scientific Results of the German Spacelab Mission D1, Norderney 1986, pp. 525–536 (WPF c/o DFVLR, Köln 1987).

Mittelstaedt, H.; Fricke, E.: The relative effect of saccular and somatosensory information on spatial perception and control Adv. Oto-Rhino-Laryng. *42:* 24–30 (Karger, Basel 1988).

Oman, C.M.; Lichtenberg, B.K.; Money, K.E.; McCoy, R.K.: MIT Canadian vestibular experiments on the Spacelab-1 mission. 4. Space motion sickness: symptoms, stimuli, and predictability. Exp. Brain Res. *64:* 316–334 (1986).

Prof. Dr. H. Mittelstaedt, Max-Planck-Institut für Verhaltensphysiologie, D-8130 Seewiesen, Post Starnberg (FRG)

Adv. Oto-Rhino-Laryng., vol. 42, pp. 24–30 (Karger, Basel 1988)

The Relative Effect of Saccular and Somatosensory Information on Spatial Perception and Control

Horst Mittelstaedt, Evi Fricke

Max-Planck-Institut für Verhaltensphysiologie, Seewiesen, FRG

This contribution deals with the role of the Z-axis component of the gravity vector, that is, the force component acting in the direction of the long axis of the head and body. Among the organs of the vestibular system, it is mainly the saccule which responds to the amount and sign of this component of the gravity vector. But clearly, many other mechanoreceptors outside the labyrinth are also affected by it.

Three problems present themselves: (1) What is the function of this information? (2) Which of these organs are involved? (3) How is their output processed?

As to function, the Z-axis gravity information has been shown [Mittelstaedt, 1983, 1985] to serve: (1) the processing of the apparent visual vertical (SV), and (2) the perception and control of body posture.

(1) The first may be demonstrated on the human centrifuge, where the subject is oriented in such a way that only the Z-axis component is modulated by the centrifugal force. As seen in figure 1, the subject is strapped, right ear down, to a padded board. In total darkness, the centrifuge is subliminally accelerated to 0.6 Hz, and the subject is asked to set a luminous pendulum to apparent vertical. The pendulum (not seen in fig. 1) may be rotated by remote control in a fronto-parallel plane about the subject's visual axis. The board with the subject and the display may be shifted radially over the horizontal platform of the centrifuge. This way, with the centrifuge axis (CA) vertical, the Z-axis of the subject is always kept normal to the earth's gravity vector and in intersection with the CA. In this orientation, the distance, d_1, of the otoliths to the CA can be varied along the Z-axis by $\pm$ 50 cm. Thereby the force acting on those otolith receptors which respond to the Z-axis force

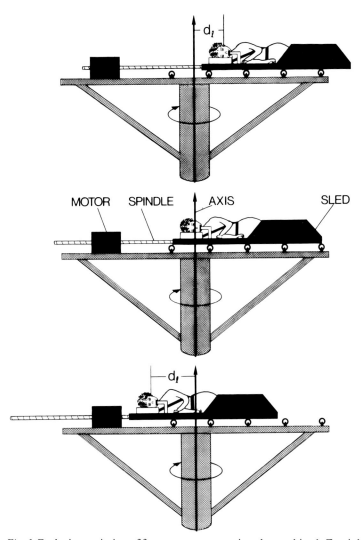

Fig. 1. Exclusive variation of force component acting along subject's Z-axis by means of human centrifuge with vertical axis and mobile horizontal platform. For testing the SV, a luminous pendulum display (not shown, but see figure 2) may be rotated about S's visual axis.

component, that is, largely those of the saccules, at a constant rotation velocity $f = 0.6$ Hz ($\omega = 3.77$ rad/s), is modulated from zero to plus or minus 0.75 g, whereas the force acting on the receptors which are sensitive to

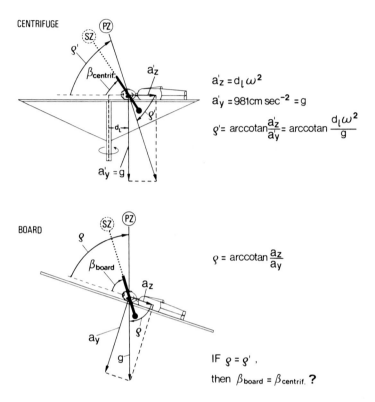

Fig. 2. Comparison of SV when the same roll angle ($\rho = \rho'$) of the force vector is produced by gravity on a tilted board (lower pictograph) or by resultant with centrifugal force (upper pictograph). SZ=Subjective zenith, PZ=physical zenith, both re head coordinates. β-Angle between pendulum and S's Z-axis. For other symbols see text.

the Y-axis force component, including those of the utricles, stays constant. When the subject is placed as shown in figure 2, the subject experiences an upward tilt. If that is due to the otoliths, we may compute the angle ρ' between the subject's Z-axis and the resultant gravito-inertial vector acting on the otoliths as:

$$\rho' = \text{arccotan}\,\frac{a'_y}{a'_z} = \text{arccotan}\,\frac{d_l\,\omega^2}{g},$$

where d_l is the distance from the eardrums to the CA, and $a'_{y/z}$ is the linear acceleration in the direction of the respective axis. Since we know that the

Table I. Extravestibular effect of caudally directed centrifugal force on SV at $d_i = 0$ (2nd column) and on subjective horizontal position with variation of ρ (3rd column) or d_i (4th column), respectively

Subject	SV at $d_1 = 0$ $\beta_i\text{-}\beta_0$ $f_i = 0.6$ Hz $f_0 = 0.0$ Hz, degrees	Self-adopted horizontal position	
		roll tilt of board ρ, degrees	distance labyr.-rot. axis d_1, cm
S.W.	+4.1 ± 2.7	91.1 ± 1.6	−11.0 ± 2.5
M.M.	+3.6 ± 1.7	92.6 ± 1.3	−8.7 ± 2.6
C.K.	+2.7 ± 2.3	88.7 ± 1.4	−26.4 ± 3.3
U.B.	+2.2 ± 4.1	89.0 ± 0.7	−12.8 ± 2.0
R.W.	+1.2 ± 6.9	90.6 ± 0.6	−30.6 ± 0.4
E.F.	+0.1 ± 2.9	92.9 ± 0.6	−3.5 ± 1.8
W.H.	−1.1 ± 1.1	91.1 ± 1.1	−25.9 ± 3.3
H.D.		88.6 ± 2.5	−50.4 ± 3.2
M.U.	−0.3 ± 5.3	85.6 ± 1.7	−39.5 ± 3.0
J.S.	−1.5 ± 5.0	92.6 ± 0.6	−42.9 ± 1.4

2nd column: difference between angle β_i at centrifuge frequency $f_i = 0.6$ Hz and angle β_0 at $f_0 = 0$. All symbols as in figure 2. All values ± SD. Last 3 S's are labyrinthine defective.

static output of the otoliths is a function of these accelerations, we may test the role of the saccule by putting the subject now on a tiltable board which is tilted by the same angle ($\rho = \rho'$; see lower part of fig. 2). Again the subject is asked to rotate, in otherwise total darkness, a luminous pendulum display via remote control until it appears vertical.

Typical examples of the results have been published in figures 5 and 6 of Mittelstaedt [1985]. If any, there are only small differences between the settings β of the pendulum in the two experiments. Such differences are to be expected at ρ, $\rho' \neq 90°$ due to the well-known saccular non-linearities; but the scatter of the settings does not allow one to identify them. At any rate, when the CA leads through the eardrums (at $\rho' = 90°$), the SV is independent of centrifuge frequency (table I, column 2). Hence the SV is indeed processed by means of otolithic, that is largely saccular, Z-axis information.

(2) It is not a matter of course that this is also true for the second function of the Z-axis information, namely the control of body posture. On the contrary, the apparent orientation of the visual world and that of one's body to the vertical are not only different phenomenally, but also mediated

by different information processing structures. Hence specific evidence about the role of the saccule is necessary.

The same apparatus and the same rationale is employed as in the first two experiments. However, with the pendulum removed, the subject is asked to change its distance d_1 from the CA or the roll angle ρ of the tiltable board, until she/he feels to lie completely horizontal. Although the subjects unanimously experience this task as much more difficult than setting the pendulum vertically and, in contrast to the latter, feel rather doubtful about their achievement, their SD turns out to be smaller (up to three times) than in the case of the SV, and their tilt close to $\rho = 90°$ on the board. And there is another surprise: as seen in table I, only one subject (E.F.) behaves on the centrifuge as expected from the result on the board *under the assumption that the self-adopted horizontal posture is achieved by means of otolith information*. All others feel to be horizontal when the CA is *caudad* of the eardrums, up to more than 30 cm, at distances d_1 which vary greately in*tra*personally, but are rather constant in*ter*personally. In 3 labyrinthine defective subjects (H.D. clinically without vestibular reactions; M.U., J.S. after bilateral section of VIIIth nerve) d_1 is found around −45 cm. There is no doubt, then, that, in contrast to the SV, extravestibular mechanoreceptors play an important part in the control of posture, and that they are situated somewhere below the head in the body.

(3) As a consequence of this result, we are now in search of the source of this additional information. A definite answer cannot yet be given, but some possible agents can be excluded. As illustrated by the pictographs inset into figure 3, the leg posture and the support forces during centrifugation have been modified. In the standard configuration (used also above), the subject is situated as if sitting on a chair and then rolled to $\rho = 90°$, that is, supported against the centrifugal force at the buttocks, thighs, and soles. In the two others, the legs are straight, such that the centrifugal force either presses them against a vertical board or stretches them out freely, with the trunk supported by mountaineer's straps.

Again the subjects are asked to manoeuvre themselves into their apparent horizontal posture. It turns out firstly that there is no difference in d_1 between the two straight-legged configurations. Hence, rather unexpectedly, leg tension or pressure does not influence postural control under these conditions. Secondly, d_1 is considerably larger in the 'extended' than in the 'bent' configuration, independent of the size of d_1, that is, even (or rather more so) in the subject (E.F.) who evinces no somatosensory influence in the bent posture.

In fact, d_1 is then much larger than expected under the assumption that the somatosensory mechanism tends to shift the CA *into the centroid of the entire*

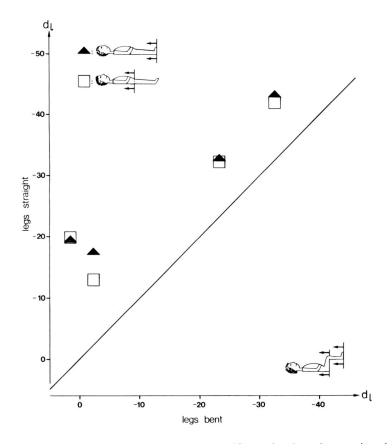

Fig. 3. Distance d_l of eardrum from centrifuge axis adopted to attain subjective horizontal position in 3 different configurations of support forces. d_l when legs are straight (▲: standing; □: mountaineer-strapped) is plotted over d_l when legs are bent (sitting), in 4 S's.

body mediated by the shear and pressure on the skin. Hence this explanation must be ruled out, at least in this strict formulation. Alternatively, it seems plausible to assume that an extended (normally 'erect') body posture enhances the influence of the somatosensory relative to that of the vestibular system. This leaves us still with the question of the former's origin. Planned experiments will test the influence of pressure receptors between the vertebrae and, lastly, of abdominal organs (as, for instance, the kidneys) transmitted by proprioceptors within their mesenteries.

References

Mittelstaedt, H.: A new solution to the problem of the subjective vertical. Naturwissen-
    schaften 70: 272–281 (1983).
Mittelstaedt, H.: Subjective vertical in weightlessness; in Igarashi, Proc. 7th Int. Symp. on
    Posture and Equilibrium, Houston 1983, pp. 139–150 (Karger, Basel 1985).

Prof. Dr. H. Mittelstaedt, Max-Planck-Institut für Verhaltensphysiologie,
D-8130 Seewiesen, Post Starnberg (FRG)

Adv. Oto-Rhino-Laryng., vol. 42, pp. 31–35 (Karger, Basel 1988)

Caloric Testing of the Vestibular Function during Orbital Flight

A.H. Clarke, H. Scherer

Department of Otorhinolaryngology, Steglitz Medical Center,
Freie Universität Berlin, West Berlin

Introduction

During the course of this century, the so-called caloric test has become invaluable in both clinical diagnosis and basic research as a method of examining the function of the vestibular system.

According to the widely accepted thermoconvective theory, as first proposed by Bárány [1] at the beginning of this century, the anisotropic changes in density resulting from thermal conduction into the temporal bone is presumed to cause convective circulation of the endolymph around the membranous duct, primarily of the horizontal semicircular canal. In turn, the hair cells enveloped by the cupula are stimulated and the afferent signal to the central vestibular system is observed to elicit an ocular reflex, as is the case during physiological angular movement of the head.

Prior to the performance of the caloric experiment in the weightlessness of orbital flight, it was generally accepted that the thermoconvective hypothesis concurred with most findings. Accordingly, it was expected that during caloric stimulation in zero-g, no convective forces would be developed and the ampullary receptors should remain unstimulated. This assumption was supported by a number of previous reports. For example, caloric experiments performed in parabolic flight [7] have demonstrated that ongoing caloric nystagmus vanishes at the onset of zero-g. However, as has been pointed out, e.g. by Jongkees [6], an immediate disappearance of the response (<1–2 s) cannot be attributed to a fluid mechanism in the canal. Rather, this effect must be attributed to a suppression mechanism in the central vestibular system of the canal-induced response, possibly by the gravity-sensitive otolith response.

In the light of these contradictory findings, the question still remained open as to whether the convective hypothesis in its generally accepted form could be upheld.

Methods

Caloric vestibular testing was performed in extended orbital flight as part of the ESA vestibular research program coordinated by von Baumgarten [2]. Central to the equipment used during both missions was the so-called 'vestibular helmet', an integrated stimulation and measurement system designed specifically for vestibular testing in the rugged environment of spaceflight.

Since for obvious reasons the use of water irrigation was prohibited during weightlessness, caloric stimulation was presented by means of air insufflation. During the first mission (SL1) bilateral stimulation was employed, with one ear stimulated above, and the other below body temperature. This mode was employed to increase the intrinsically lower intensity of stimulation with air insufflation. During the second mission (D1), unilateral stimulation was also employed.

Recording of the caloric nystagmus response was performed by means of horizontal and vertical electro-oculographic recording (EOG). In addition, an infrared-sensitive video camera was mounted in front of the left eye for online monitoring and digital image processing of eye movements. The ESA vestibular sled, which was flown on the D1 mission, provided precise linear acceleratory stimulation. The acceleration profile employed for the caloric experiment involved a sled displacement of ± 1.6 m, with sinusoidal acceleration along the anterior-posterior axis with peak values of 100 or 200 mg.

Preflight baseline data collection was performed at regular intervals during astronaut training. Postflight measurements were carried out directly after landing and continued over a period of 12 days.

Results

Caloric nystagmus was observed in both tested subjects during the 7-day Spacelab-SL1 mission. Full details have been reported elsewhere by Scherer et al. [10]. Summarily, the SL1 findings showed that: (1) the inflight zero-g responses were in all respects comparable to those measured on ground in one-g conditions, (2) further, the direction of the nystagmus was always consistent with the stimulus presented and reversed promptly after inversion of the temperature gradient.

Whereas the first experiment series was performed primarily to examine the adequacy of Bárány's thermoconvection theory, it was intended during the subsequent D1 mission to examine the effect of linear acceleratory stimulation on an ongoing caloric nystagmus.

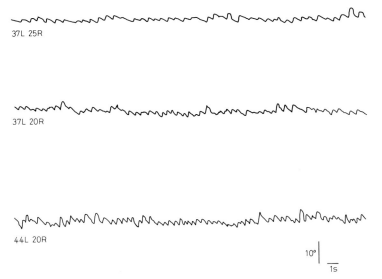

37L 25R

37L 20R

44L 20R

10° |
‾‾‾
1s

Fig. 1. Examples of caloric nystagmus recorded during the D1 mission. (Contrary to normal convention eye movement to the right is represented by downward deflection on the tracing.) The first two examples, for stimulus temperatures of 37L/25R and 37L/25R represent unilateral stimulation. The third pair 44L/15R represents a bilateral stimulation. It can be observed that the intensity of the nystagmus (as described by the SPV and frequency) increases with the differential temperature – whether unilateral or bilateral.

During this mission the caloric stimulation was performed on a total of 3 subjects, repeated tests being carried out on 2 of them. Tests were performed on days 0, 2, 5 and 6 of the mission. Nystagmus response to the caloric stimulus was observed in all tests performed during the mission (fig. 1).

Analysis of the data from sled runs during caloric stimulation performed in early flight shows that a clear modulation of nystagmus activity occurs during linear acceleration along the anterior-posterior axis. Indeed, it appears that the polarity of the observed nystagmus could be switched according to whether positive or negative acceleratory stimulation were applied (fig. 2). During the phases of negative-going X-axis acceleration (in which the direction of the acceleration vector corresponds with the face-up, supine position in the one-*g* environment) the original nystagmus direction is maintained. However, it appears that during the phases of positive-going X-axis acceleration (which would correspond to the face-down, prone position in one-*g*) an inversion of the ongoing nystagmus is accomplished.

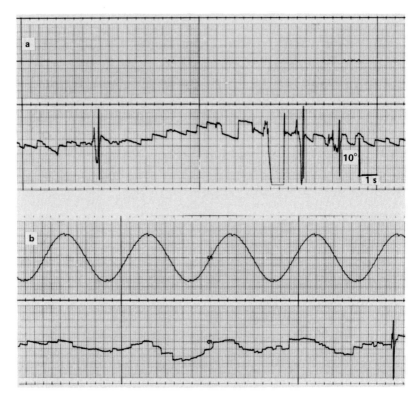

Fig. 2. Nystagmus modulation during sled acceleration. Upper trace, sled acceleration; lower trace, horizontal EOG: *a* response while sled stationary, *b* response during sinusoidal sled acceleration run (200 mG).

Discussion

The findings from both the SL1 and D1 experiments demonstrate that – after initial adaptation – the caloric nystagmus elicited in the microgravity conditions of extended orbital flight is equivalent to that observed in one-*g* earthbound testing. These findings clearly demonstrate the inadequacy of any thesis which rests solely on the idea of a thermoconvective mechanism in the inner ear. Of the possible alternative mechanisms, which might be responsible for this 'zero-*g*' nystagmus, the present authors would favor those hypotheses based, firstly, on direct thermally mediated volume shifts in the ampullofugal and ampullopetal directions around the endolymph duct and, secondly, on the thermal influence on the end organ and nerve endings in the ampullae [9].

Whilst it is possible that the observed modulation of nystagmus response by linear acceleration is caused by the generation of a convective torque during sled acceleration, we would prefer to associate it with those reports on otolith-canal interaction processes in the central vestibular system related to the concept of velocity storage. Comparable examples have been reported on the modification of the caloric response by linear acceleration [3], the modification of optokinetic nystagmus by linear acceleration [4], and the modulation of off-vertical axis rotatory nystagmus by the otolith input to central storage mechanisms [5, 8].

References

1 Bárány, R.: Untersuchungen über den vom Vestibularapparat des Ohres reflektorisch ausgelösten rhythmischen Nystagmus und seine Begleiterscheinungen. Mschr. Ohrenheilk. *40:* 193–297 (1906).
2 Baumgarten, R. von; Benson, A.; Berthoz, A.; Brandt, T.; Brandt, U.; Bruzek, W.; Dichgans, J.; Kass, J.; Probst, T.; Scherer, H.; Viéville, T.; Vogel, H.; Wetzig, J.: Effects of rectilinear acceleration and optokinetic and caloric stimulation in space. The spacelab experience: a synopsis. Science *225:* 208–212 (1984).
3 Benson, A.: Modification of the response to angular accelerations by linear accelerations; in Kornhuber, Handbook of sensory physiology, vol. VI/2, pp. 282–320 (Springer, Berlin 1974).
4 Buizza, A.; Leger, A.; Droulez, J.; Berthoz, A.; Schmid, R.: Influence of otolithic stimulation by horizontal linear acceleration on optokinetic nystagmus and visual motor perception. Exp. Brain Res. *39:* 165–176 (1980).
5 Harris, L.R.: The effect of opposing and otolith signals during off-vertical-axis rotation in the cat. J. Physiol. *371:* 30P (1986),
6 Jongkees, L.B.W.: Physiologie und Pathophysiologie des Vestibularorganes. Arch. klin. exp. Ohr.-Nas.-KehlkHeilk. *194:* 1–110 (1969).
7 Kellogg, R.S.; Graybiel, A.: Lack of response to thermal stimulation of the semicircular canals in the weightless phase of parabolic flight. Aerospace Med. *38:* 487–490 (1967).
8 Raphan, T.; Matsuo, V.; Cohen, B.: Effects of gravity on rotatory nystagmus in monkeys; in Cohen, Vestibular and oculomotor physiology. Ann. N.Y. Acad. Sci. *374:* 337–346 (1981).
9 Scherer, H.; Clarke, A.H.: The caloric vestibular reaction in space. Physiological considerations. Acta oto-lar. *100:* 328–336 (1985).
10 Scherer, H.; Clarke, A.H.; Brandt, U.; Merbold, U.; Parker, R.: Caloric nystagmus in microgravity. European vestibular experiments in the Spacelab-1 mission. Exp. Brain Res. *64:* 255–263 (1986).

Dr. A.H. Clarke, HNO-Klinik, Klinikum Steglitz, Hindenburgdamm 30, D-1000 Berlin 45 (FRG)

Adv. Oto-Rhino-Laryng., vol. 42, pp. 36–38 (Karger, Basel 1988)

Eye Movements Induced by Calorization of the Vertical Semicircular Canals. A Study in Pigeon

H.A.A. de Jong, H.P. Goossens, W.J. Oosterveld

Vestibular Department ENT, University of Amsterdam, The Netherlands

Introduction

The appearance of caloric nystagmus in man during orbital flight in Spacelab [1] caused a revival of the discussion around its explanation. Ewald [2] found differences between horizontal and vertical labyrinthine reflex responses after rotation stimulation. At least two canals, one on each side, are simultaneously affected by a rotatory stimulus. This study deals with eye movement patterns in pigeon resulting from stimulation on one vertical canal.

Methods

Fifteen pigeons were subjected to 361 vertical semicircular canal calorizations in ground-based conditions. Five pigeons were exposed to 184 parabolic manoeuvres of an airplane (Fokker F-27). They were subjected 48 times to the caloric test during microgravity and submitted 60 times to the tests during higher g-load conditions. Only a particular circumscribed part of a labyrinth was stimulated by a minor temperature change by a special technique [3, 4].

The stimulation parts of the vertical semicircular canal were respectively chosen at the most posterior and the most lateral descending curve of the canal. Minor pressure changes in a syringe resulted in a constant temperature at the selected site of the canal within a variation of 0.2 °C. The optimal responses were obtained by a temperature difference of 2 °C above or below body temperature.

Results

'Internal calorization' of one of the four vertical semicircular canals evoked vertical nystagmus. The intensity and the slow phase velocity proved to be proportional to the magnitude of the temperature difference between both labyrinths (fig. 1).

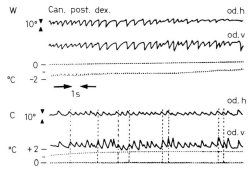

Fig. 1. Horizontal and vertical movement of the right eye in pigeon during cold (C) and warm (W) calorization of the canalis posterior dexter. Change of temperature from −2 to +2 °C (0 °C=body temperature) causes an inversion of both vertical and horizontal nystagmus. Mind desynchronization of the horizontal and vertical eye movements in lower graph. The induced movements of the left eye are similar but opposite directed as compared to the horizontal and vertical movements of the right eye. od.h = horizontal movement of the right eye; od.v.=vertical movement of the right eye.

During cold calorization a slow phase velocity up (upper graph) and during warm calorization a slow phase velocity downwards (lower graph) showed up. To these movements a weaker horizontal component was added. During cold calorization this slow phase velocity horizontal was directed ipsilaterally and during warm calorization contralaterally.

With the plane of the stimulated vertical canal perpendicular to the direction of gravity, this calorization did not cause any eye deviation. However, during sustained stimulation the vertical eye movements showed up again when this canal was turned back in the vertical plane (animal in prone position).

Besides the position dependency of the eye movements, a gravity dependency showed up. The vertical nystagmus induced by vertical canal calorization disappeared during shortlasting weightless periods [5–7]. The nystagmus raised up again and increased proportional to the gravitational force a few seconds after the onset of the gravity.

Discussion

Suggestions are made that expansion or contraction of the endolymph and peri-ectolymph fluids during warm and cold calorization could affect the cupula [1]. However, Paige [8] reported an unchangeable horizontal slow phase velocity directed to the irrigated side after blockade of the stimulated horizontal canal in the face-up or face-down position. He explained the phenomenon by a direct thermal effect on the sensory nerve endings [9]. During warm horizontal canal calorization both a direct thermal effect and the expansion influence will combine their action in modifying the final rate of the afferent discharge of the sensory cells of the cupula that is stimulated by convection during warm or cold calorization. This situation is different during vertical canal calorization. Regardless of the position of the cupula, under or above the stimulated site of the vertical canal, during cold and warm calorization, the direct thermal effect and the influence of expansion or contraction will act in opposite directions to each other.

In view of these combined and concerting actions of the direct thermal effect and expansion influence during external canal calorization, and their opposing actions during vertical canal calorization, we explain the vestibular caloric nystagmus during orbital flight in Spacelab as a part of the total central vestibular habituation, instead of these peripheral vestibular influences.

References

1   Scherer, H.; Clarke, A.H.: The caloric vestibular reaction in space. Acta oto-lar. *100:* 328–336 (1985)
2   Ewald, J.R.: Physiologische Untersuchungen über das Endorgan des N. Oktavus (Bergmann, Wiesbaden 1982).
3   Gursel, A.O.; Jong, H.A.A. de; Oosterveld, W.J.: Internal and external vestibular caloric test in pigeons. A nystagmographic study. ORL *45:* 270–278 (1983).
4   Jong, H.A.A. de; Goossens, H.P.; Oosterveld, W.J.: Vertical nystagmus provoked by locally applied calorization at the vertical semi-circular canals. A study in pigeon. ORL (in press, 1988).
5   Oosterveld, W.J.; Laarse, W.D. van der: Effect of gravity on vestibular nystagmus. Aerospace Med. *40:* 382–385 (1969).
6   Oosterveld, W.J.; Greven, A.J.; Gursel, A.O.; Jong, H.A.A. de: Caloric vestibular test in the weightless phase of parabolic flight. Acta oto-lar. *99:* 571–576 (1985).
7   Graybiel, A.; O'Donnell, R.D.; Fluur, E.; Nagaba, M.; Smith, M.J.: Mechanisms underlying modulations of thermal nystagmic responses in parabolic flight. Acta oto-lar. suppl. 378, pp. 1–16 (1980).
8   Paige, G.D.: .Caloric responses after horizontal canal inactivation. Acta oto-lar. *100:* 321–327 (1985).
9   Coats, A.C.; Smith, S.Y.: Body position and the intensity of caloric nystagmus. Acta oto-lar. *63:* 515–532 (1967).

H.A.A. de Jong, MD, University of Amsterdam, Academisch Medisch Centrum, Vestibular Department, Meibergdreef 9, NL-1105 AZ Amsterdam
(The Netherlands)

Adv. Oto-Rhino-Laryng., vol. 42, pp. 39–42 (Karger, Basel 1988)

Inner Ear Blood Flow in the Rabbit after Caloric Stimulation[1]

C. Angelborg, H.C. Larsen, G. Levin

University Hospital, Uppsala, Sweden

Introduction

The convection theory of caloric induced nystagmus [Barany, 1906] has been generally accepted. However, recent results obtained during flight in space cannot be explained using this theory. In microgravity nystagmus has been elicited with comparable intensity to that of preflight and postflight examinations [Scherer and Clarke, 1985]. Neither does the convection theory explain the observation that the caloric response is greater in the supine position than when elicited with the head in the prone position [Barany, 1907].

The mode in which the vestibular organ reacts to caloric stimuli is not fully understood and new theories have been proposed; among others the possibility of a direct temperature effect on the endorgan [Coats and Smith, 1967] has been proposed. The current study was made to find out whether any caloric vestibular response can be mediated by changes in inner ear blood flow.

Material and Methods

Ten healthy male albino rabbits with a body weight between 1.5 and 2.0 kg were used. The microspheres used in the present study were carbonized latex particles radioactively labelled with ^{141}Ce or ^{87}Sr. They had a diameter of 9.0 ± 0.5 μm (3M, Minn., USA) and were dissolved in saline with Tween® and ultrasonicated before injection; 1.5 ml containing about 20×10^6 microspheres was used at each injection.

The animals were anesthetized with intravenously administered sodium pentotal (50–60 mg/kg body weight) before surgery. When necessary the anesthesia was

[1] This work was supported by grants from the Swedish Medical Research Council, No. 17X–04782.

supported with 1% lidocain locally for tracheotomy and catheterization of the femoral arteries. After the tracheostomy the animals were artificially ventilated in a respirator (excessor bag).

Body temperature was kept constant by a heating pad and polyethylene catheters were induced into each femoral artery, one for continuous blood pressure measurements and the other for reference blood sampling. After thoracotomy a catheter was placed in the left ventricle of the heart through which the arterial acid base balance was controlled and the microsphere injection performed.

When the arterial acid base balance was found to be within normal range the first microsphere injection was made over 10 s and the reference blood sample was simultaneously collected for 60 s. Thereafter, cold water (0 °C) was injected into the left ear canal for 30 s at a pressure of 15 kPa. After 2 min the next microsphere injection was performed with microspheres labelled with another isotope. A reference blood sample was collected as described above.

Within 2 min the animals were killed with intracardially injected saturated KC1. The animals were decapitated and the temporal bones removed. After microdissection the radioactivity was measured in the cochlea, the vestibular parts of the inner ear and the reference blood samples. The blood flow was calculated by the equation:

$$f_0 = n_0 \times f_{ref}/n_{ref},$$

where f_0=the blood flow in the part investigated, n_0=the radioctivity of the part investigated, f_{ref}=the amount of reference blood, and n_{ref}=the radioactivity in the reference blood sample. Students t-test for paired comparison was used for the statistical calculation and all results are expressed as $\bar{x} \pm SD$.

Results

All animals tolerated the anesthesia, surgery and microsphere injection well. During and after the injection of cold water the animals exhibited nystagmus. The MAP and acid base balance did not differ between the first and second blood flow measurements (table I). In 5 of the 10 animals the cochlear blood flow increased slightly but not significantly after the caloric stimulation (table II). In 2 of the animals there was a slight decrease of the vestibular blood flow after the caloric stimulation but in all other experiments the vestibular and cochlear blood flow did not react with any correlation to the caloric stimulation.

Discussion

In order to test the role of convection of inner ear fluids in the caloric reaction, Paige [1985] plugged the horizontal canal. The convection current was thereby abolished but still there was a response seen from the plugged ear

Table I. Mean arterial pressure and acid base balance before (1) and after (2) caloric stimulation

No	MAP kPa		PCO$_2$ kPa		PO$_2$ kPa		pH	
	(1)	(2)	(1)	(2)	(1)	(2)	(1)	(2)
1	11	11	2.61	2.67	13.4	13.2	7.42	7.41
2	12	12	3.45	3.97	12.5	11.2	7.41	7.36
3	12	12	3.42	3.69	13.0	11.9	7.53	7.50
4	12	12	4.39	3.97	9.8	9.9	7.46	7.47
5	12	12	4.15	4.34	10.4	10.0	7.51	7.46
6	10	10	3.73	3.29	8.9	9.5	7.35	7.33
7	11	10	4.62	3.47	13.0	12.7	7.54	7.54
8	11	10	3.51	4.66	9.6	10.46	7.45	7.37
9	12	12	4.42	4.18	8.2	8.7	7.54	7.53
10	10	10	2.74	2.82	13.0	10.7	7.47	7.48
(1)	11.3±0.78		3.70±0.66		11.2±1.89		7.47±0.06	
(2)	11.1±0.94		3.71±0.61		10.8±1.36		7.46±0.07	

Table II. Cochlear and vestibular blood flow before (1) and after (2) caloric stimulation

No.	Cochlear blod flow, mg/min				Vestibular blood flow, mg/min			
	(1)		(2)		(1)		(2)	
	right	left	right	left	right	left	right	left
1	3.32	3.54	2.64	2.66	1.43	1.32	1.05	1.07
2	3.44	5.65	2.74	4.34	1.64	2.13	1.07	1.54
3	4.93	3.70	5.18	3.90	1.35	1.03	1.98	1.15
4	3.96	3.76	4.30	3.87	1.61	1.83	1.86	1.76
5	5.79	3.16	5.87	3.71	1.68	2.29	1.99	2.16
6	2.75	2.90	2.54	2.70	1.11	1.25	1.30	1.42
7	3.34	3.75	2.94	3.12	1.87	1.93	1.56	1.78
8	3.02	3.18	3.10	2.60	1.17	1.51	1.06	1.98
9	1.54	1.40	1.50	1.60	0.83	0.97	0.82	0.86
10	1.08	0.65	1.89	0.85	0.34	0.50	0.57	0.88
right	3.31±1.33		3.27±1.33		1.30±04.4		1.33±0.47	
left	3.16±1.30		2.94±1.04		1.48±0.54		1.46±0.44	

with the direction of the nystagmus contralaterally irrespective of head position. A direct temperature effect on the endorgan in vestibular response was estimated to be almost one third of that of the effect of the convection current. A third factor of unclear origin was found.

Scherer and Clarke [1985] suggested a volume displacement as the cause of the caloric reaction. Theoretically, this could be a vascular reaction by a direct change in blood cirulation. A temperature-induced change of inner ear fluid volume, of which the blood in the vessels makes up a considerable part, will bring about a displacement of the cupula. Such displacement may explain the eliciting of nystagmus in microgravity and also the reactions from a plugged canal.

In the present investigation there were no indications of any change of the inner ear blood flow. If there is a direct volume displacement, this does not seem to influence the blood circulation.

References

Alm, A.; Bill, A.: The oxygen supply to the retina. II. Effects of high intraocular pressure on uveal and retinal blood flow in the cat. A study with labelled microspheres including flow determinations in brain and some other tissues. Acta physiol. scand. *84:* 306–319 (1972).

Angelborg, C.; Larsen, H.C.: Blood flow in the peripheral vestibular system. J. Otolaryngol. *14:* 41–43 (1985).

Bárány, R.: Untersuchungen über den vom Vestibularisapparat des Ohres reflektorisch ausgelösten Nystagmus und seine Begleiterscheinungen. Mschr. Ohrenheilk. *40:* 193–297 (1906).

Bárány, R.: Physiologie und Pathologie (Funktionsprüfung) des Bogengang-Apparates beim Menschen (Deuticke, Leipzig 1907).

Carlborg, C.: On physiological and experimental variations of the perilymphatic pressure in the cat. Acta oto-lar. *91:* 19–28 (1981).

Coats, A.C.; Smith, S.Y.: Body position and the intensity of caloric nystagmus. Acta oto-lar. *63:* 515–532 (1967).

Hultcrantz, E.; Larsen, H.C.; Angelborg, A.: Effects of CO_2 inhalation on cochlear blood circulation. ORL *42:* 304–312 (1980).

Paige, G.D.: Caloric responses after horizontal canal inactivation. Acta oto-lar. *100:* 321–327 (1985).

Scherer, H.; Clarke, A.H.: The caloric vestibular reaction in space. Acta oto-lar. *100:* 328–336 (1985).

C. Angelborg, MD, University Hospital Uppsala, S-75185 Uppsala (Sweden)

Adv. Oto-Rhino-Laryng., vol. 42, pp. 43–49 (Karger, Basel 1988)

Objective and Quantitative Vestibular Spinal Testing by Means of Computer-Video-Cranio-Corpo-Graphy

C.-F. Claussen, E. Claussen

Neurootological Research Institute of the 4-G-F e.V., Bad Kissingen, FRG

Introduction

Modern equilibriometry is dealing with objectively and quantitatively recording and measuring human equilibrium functions. Besides the oculomotor movements, i.e. nystagmus, the head and body movements are increasingly of interest to the clinician dealing with patients suffering from vertigo, dizziness, instability and gait disorders.

Nearly 20 years ago cranio-corpo-graphy was designed as a non-electronic, simple office recording procedure for head and body movements. The light tracings of the head and shoulder movements are transformed, through an instant camera, into photographs which look like a radar image of the head and shoulders floating in space. This set of tests especially was developed for the West German Berufsgenossenschaften (labour security surveillance boards) as a field test for occupational medical purposes. In 1983 it was officially introduced into occupational medicine in the FRG through the decree G 41 of the West German Berufsgenossenschaften.

For achieving an on-line automatic measurement of the main parameters of the head and shoulder movements we have further developed cranio-corpo-graphy towards the computer-video-cranio-corpo-graphy (CVCCG).

Materials and Methods

Basically, CVCCG uses the same principle as the conventional cranio-corpo-graphy for recording the vestibular spinal reactions of the head and shoulders photo-optically. The patient is marked by means of a workman's hard hat containing light bulbs above the forehead and the occiput and cables with connecting light bulbs for both shoulders. A battery, a circuit and a switch are kept within the helmet. For excluding optic stimuli the patient is blindfolded by means of a sleeping mask.

Regularly the test procedure contains 2 different tests. Firstly we use the very sensitive stepping test (Unterberger, Fukuda). During the test the patient has to make 80–100 steps on the spot optimally during 1 min. After about 30–40 steps the patient has mostly lost or reduced his remembered space orientation so that he is depending much more on the inertia forces acting on his vestibular inner ear system for orientation.

The 4 important parameters for quantitatively evaluating the stepping test cranio-corpo-grams are: (1) longitudinal displacement from the starting to the end position in cm; (2) lateral sway width during the stepping cycles measured in cm; (3) the angular deviation in degrees between the direction of the starting position towards the connecting line with the end position; (4) the body axis spin in angular degrees in the end position with respect to the starting position.

The second test being used is the standing test procedure (Romberg). The patient is requested to stand upright with the feet close together during 1–3 min. This test is very rigid. It depends much on the function of proprioception of the cerebellum and supratentorial sections of the brain. The main parameters for evaluating this test are: (1) the longitudinal sway in cm; (2) the lateral sway in cm; (3) the torticollis angle in degree of the cranial torque with respect to the axis of the shoulders.

Instead of using the conventional instant camera above the head of the patient for the vertical projection of the head and shoulder movements, we have introduced a black and white video camera with a fish-eye lens for having the system still recording at a small distance between the camera and the headlights (fig. 1). The video image is on-line digitized and input into a small personal computer which was modified. For establishing 4 data files of the tracings of the light marks from the forehead, the occiput, the right shoulder and the left shoulder, the patient has initially to be positioned precisely under the camera, so that the 0-point data can be transferred to a special display of 4 LED. When all the 4 light-emitting diodes are switched on, this indicates that the computer program has caught the starting position of the 4 tracer lights. At this moment the test can be started. The patient is requested to begin with his stepping or standing procedure. The computer is instructed to start the recording through a push-button signal. CVCCG was developed in cooperation with the company Med-Electronic of Unterlei-nach (Würzburg). During the phase of development of this system the computer was aided by a visual CRT display signal to enable the investigator to follow directly the movements on the screen. The final system only contains the light spot catcher indicators and a 4-colour plotter. As soon as the patient leaves the range of visual surveillance of the camera with one or several of the marker lights, the representative LED are extinguished. This then leads to default indications.

The recording time for both the stepping tests and the standing tests is preset. Normally we use 1 min. Directly at the end of the investigation the computer starts calculating the 4 data files representing the points of position of the light marks from the forehead, the occiput, the right shoulder and the left shoulder.

After calculation of the representative parameters of the stepping test — i.e. (1) longitudinal displacement, (2) lateral sway, (3) angular deviation, (4) body spin — a graphical and numerical chart is plotted on the 4-colour strip chart plotter. In the upper part of this form the head and shoulder movements are graphed in a rectangular coordinate system starting from the center point. Beneath this graph a schedule is printed containing the description and the numerical values of the representative parameters. The same is performed for the standing procedure.

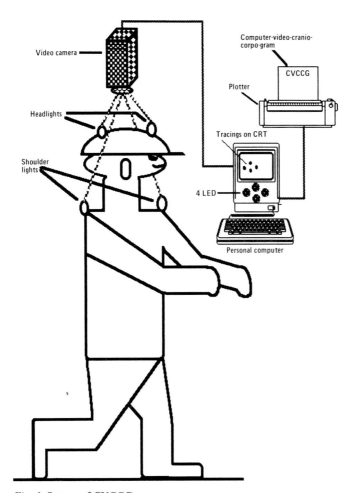

Fig. 1. Set-up of CVCCG.

Whereas the measurements of the various parameters are corrected for the optical distortion introduced through the superwide angle of the fish-eye lens. the graphical display shows non-linearly growing scales on the abscissa and the ordinate. This is necessary as the graph is not yet linearly corrected.

Examples of Typical CVCCG

The first example shows a normal case with a longitudinal displacement, a small lateral sway and no pathological lateral deviations during the stepping test procedure (fig. 2).

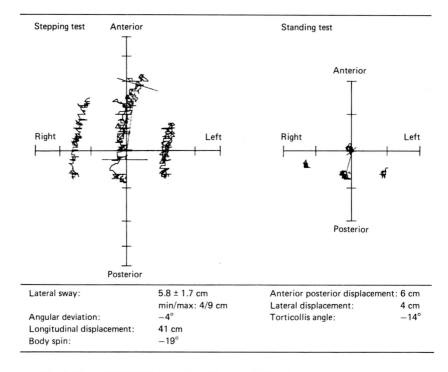

Fig. 2. Normal CVCCG, in A.P., a 16-year-old female.

The second case exhibits the typical signs of a peripheral vestibular lesion. During the stepping test the patient is significantly deviating towards the right side of the peripheral vestibular inhibition; however, the lateral sway is not enlarged beyond the limits of normality (fig. 3).

The third case demonstrates the typical pattern of a central brain stem disinhibition of the cerebello-ponto-medullary type. The size of the lateral sway lies much above the limits of normality (fig. 4).

Discussion

As the conventional photo-optical cranio-corpo-graphy has proved to be an important tool for equilibriometric field investigations, the demand for research into details and special parameters has increased. It was obvious that quantitative measurements are much easier to handle with modern

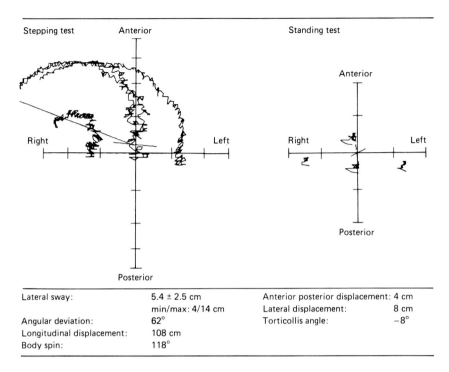

Lateral sway:	5.4 ± 2.5 cm	Anterior posterior displacement: 4 cm
	min/max: 4/14 cm	Lateral displacement: 8 cm
Angular deviation:	62°	Torticollis angle: −8°
Longitudinal displacement:	108 cm	
Body spin:	118°	

Fig. 3. CVCCG indicating a peripheral vestibular lesion on the right side, B.A., a 64-year-old male, with acute vertigo attacks of long duration, hypoacusia and hypertension.

electronic data acquisition techniques and computers. More than a year ago, in cooperation with the Med-Electronic Company of Unterleinach (Würz-burg) we started to assemble a setup of a video camera, a digitizer and a personal computer (fig. 1) for transforming the 4 different light tracings into 4 separate data files. In each file every data point contains the Cartesian coordinates as well as the time coordinate of the spatial position of the light mark. It was then easy to find the starting and ending positions. At any time interval the 4 positional points of the right shoulder, of the left shoulder, the forehead and the occiput can be charted and geometrically rectified. There-after, the direction and position can be calculated.

Thus, CVCCG continues a trend of objective recording and quantitative evaluation of head and body movements in the clinical diagnostics of disequilibrium states. An advantage of running the procedure through the video-computer combination is the possibility of introducing patient-related

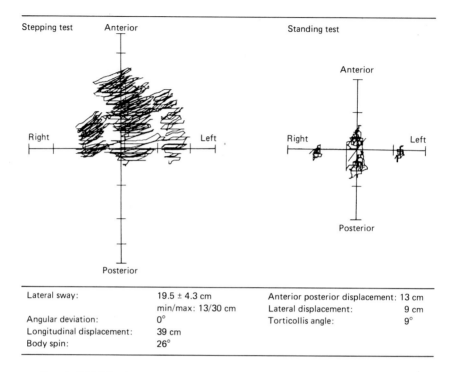

Lateral sway:	19.5 ± 4.3 cm	Anterior posterior displacement:	13 cm
	min/max: 13/30 cm	Lateral displacement:	9 cm
Angular deviation:	0°	Torticollis angle:	9°
Longitudinal displacement:	39 cm		
Body spin:	26°		

Fig. 4. CVCCG of a central disequilibrium with an enlarged lateral head and body sway, B.L., a 55-year-old female complaining of headache, vertigo, nausea, hypoacusia and hypertension.

data files into the recording. The prococol then combines personal data with a schedule of measurements and with a combined graphical and numerical form.

The results of the investigation are available very soon after performing the test. It is nearly an on-line procedure. However, when introducing the electronic and computer assembly into the objectively recorded head and body movement measurements, the whole test has become more sophisticated from the point of view of maintenance of the machinery. The increase of accuracy in the numerical evaluation and the increase in the precision of the layout of the test results in an improved clinical form is only gained by a reduction of simplicity in the apparatuses. At present we are still modifying the system. This article is therefore only a preliminary report.

References

Claussen, C.-F.: Über eine Gleichgewichtsfunktionsprüfung mit Hilfe der Cranio-Corpo-Graphie (CCG) und Polarkoordinaten im Raume. Arch. klin. exp. Ohr.-Nas.-Kehlk-Heilk. *196:* 256–261 (1970).
Claussen, C.-F.: Schwindel-Symptomatik, Diagnostik, Therapie. Edition Medicin & Pharmacie (Rudat, Hamburg 1981).
Claussen, C.-F.: Presbyvertigo, Presbyataxie, Presbytinnitus (Springer, Berlin 1985).
Claussen, C.F.; Claussen, E.: Forschungsbericht Cranio-Corpo-Graphie (CCG) — Ein einfacher, objektiver und quantitativer Gleichgewichtstest für die Praxis. Schriftenreihe des Hauptverbandes der gewerblichen Berufsgenossenschaften e.V., St. Augustin 1986.
Claussen, C.-F; Claussen, E.; Schlachta, I. von: Das impulsmarkierte Cranio-Corpo-Gramm, ein differenzierter vestibulo-spinaler Test mit besonderer Bedeutung für die Arbeitsmedizin. Neurootologie in Forschung und Praxis. Symp. über Neurootologie, Rostock 1983, pp. 117–123.
Romberg, H.: Lehrbuch der Nervenkrankheiten, pp.. 184–191 (Springer, Berlin 1848).
Unterberger, S.: Neue objektive registrierbare Vestibulariskörperdrehreaktionen, erhalten durch Treten auf der Stelle. Der Tretversuch. Arch. Ohr.-Nas-KehlkHeilk. *145:* 273–282 (1938).

Prof. Dr. Claus-F. Claussen, Extraordinarius für Neurootologie, Kurhausstrasse 12, D-8730 Bad Kissingen (FRG)

Adv. Oto-Rhino-Laryng., vol. 42, pp. 50–54 (Karger, Basel 1988)

Median Filtering of Stabilometric Data

H. Aalto[a], *I. Pyykkö*[b], *M. Juhola*[c], *J. Starck*[a]

[a]Institute of Occupational Health, Vantaa; [b]Department of Otolaryngology, University Hospital of Helsinki, Helsinki; [c]Institute of Computer Science, University of Turku, Turku, Finland.

Introduction

The dynamic range of posturography signals depends on the sensitivity of the force transducers, properties of the amplifiers and, when fed into the computer, from the properties of the analog to digital (AD) converter. If an FM-tape recorder is used for the storage of the measurements, the signal-to-noise ratio seldom exceeds 40 dB (100:1). A parameter often used to characterize body sway or stability is the line integral between two adjacent points of centerpoint of force [Kapteyn et al., 1983]. Errors generated by noise in the coordinate points mean increased length to the sway path. This can be avoided using properly filtering techniques.

As the unavoidable quantization noise from the analog to digital conversion has to be filtered in any case in digital form, additional software filtering can be easily applied. This enables the use of more powerful nonlinear algorithms in the smoothing process instead of the commonly used conventional linear filtering technique. One such possibility is the nonlinear median filter. It is known to be particularly effective in removing impulsive noise and in preserving rapid changes in signal levels [Heinonen et al., 1985]. Its especially transient elimination property is useful in eliminating short transient-like artifacts originating from tape speed alterations or other mechanical incompleteness of the tape recording process.

Median Filter

The median filter algorithm is a simple operation of choosing the median value of the samples (X1, X2, ..., Xn) inside a moving window of fixed length (n = 2k+1). By definition, the median value is both the (k+1) largest and (k+1) smallest value inside the processing window. Thus, the median filtering is principally a simple choosing operation, but when the window size is large, the process will be very time-consuming.

For filtering of posturography signal we have chosen the simplest form of median filter (k = 1) which is composed of a three-point processing window. The median datapoint inside the window gets the value which is neither the greatest nor the smallest value in magnitude. This gives the filter the property that one single data value has no meaning alone, but that two consecutive values are true. In general form it means that a transient shorter than half the length of the processing window will be eliminated. In this application short transients of one datapoint will be reduced to the level of their surrounding points, as well as transients that contain two datapoints on the opposite side of the mean value.

As the median filter uses only existing data values, a smoothing section should be added. It is realized by a moving average filter using a three-point data-processing window. This linear filter reduces, furthermore, the high frequency noise originating mainly from the quantization process. The final step is again a combination of median and moving average filtering. Tests with sinusoidal signals using a 33.3-Hz sampling rate give an approximately 50% reduction of amplitude for 4.1-Hz signal frequency.

A phenomenon called aliasing or folding can occur if the sampling rate is less than twice the highest frequency in the recorded signal. In the case of median filter, the minimal sampling frequency requirement is four times the highest signal frequency; otherwise, aliasing cannot be avoided.

Effect of Filtering in Posturography Signal

Median filtering is applied to a stabilometric recording of 175 s duration (fig. 1). Three stimulation-free conditions and 5 conditions with vibration applied to the calf muscles were analyzed [Pyykkö et al., 1986]. Sway velocity was the parameter calculated. It is the line integral of centerpoint of force coordinates divided by time. The same data are replayed and analyzed from an FM-tape recorder. Three repetitive analyses were made without filtering and subsequently three analyses with filtering. The effect of filtering on the centerpoint of force signal is shown in figure 1b. The median and max/min values obtained for sway velocity parameters without filtering and the max/min values obtained with filtering are shown in figure 2. Filtering reduced the

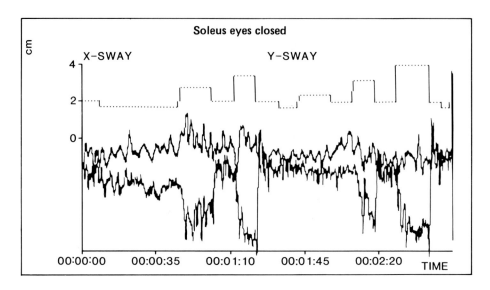

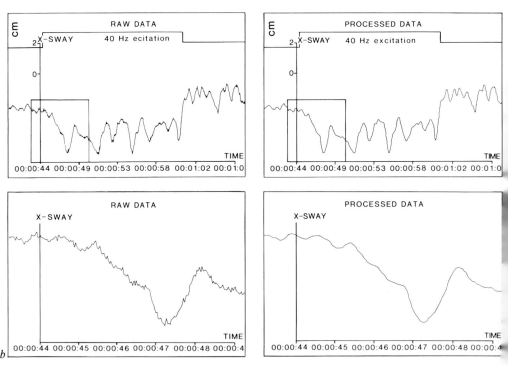

Fig. 1. a Stabilogram. Upper diagram shows vibration periods and frequencies. Middle trace is the centerpoint of force coordinates in right-left direction, and lowest trace is the centerpoint of force coordinates in fore-aft directions. *b* Enlarged graph (5 s) from the fore-aft signal of *a*.

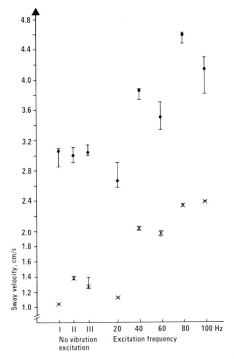

Fig. 2. Sway velocities of one measurement. Repeated analysis (n=3) from FM-recorded measurement without (dotted vertical bars) and with (crossed vertical bars) filtering. Sway velocities in background condition (bk) (30 s) and with 5 vibration stimuli applied on soleus muscles.

sway velocity values by about 65% to 1.1 cm/s which is close to the values reported by Taguchi et al. [1978], 1.4 cm/s, and by Hufschmidt et al. [1980], 1.7 cm/s. The uncertainty of the analysis is also reduced.

Conclusion

Computer-graded parameter calculation does not tolerate noise levels caused by analog tape recording processes without a significant change in a certain parameter value in body sway analysis. Conventional linear methods are suitable for eliminating quantization noise, but short transients of great magnitude will be eliminated more effectively by a simple nonlinear median filter in reasonable time. The method introduced can be applied to all data where a few adjacent data values inside a processing window of fixed length can be ignored as (random or transient) noise, and corrected to the level of its neighborhood without significantly distorting the information of the measured signal.

References

Heinonen, P.; Kalli, S.; Turjanmaa, V.; Neuvo, Y.: Generalized median filters for biological signal processing. Proc. 7th Eur. Conf. on Circuit Theory and Design, Prague 1985, pp. 283–286.

Hufschmidt, A.; Dichgans, J.; Mauritz, K.-H.; Hufschmidt, M.: Some methods and parameters of body sway quantification and their neurological applications. Archs Psychiat. neurol. Sci. *228:* 135–150 (1980).

Kapteyn, T.S.; Bles, W.; Njiokiktjien, C.J.; Kodde, L.; Massen, C.H.; Mol, J.M.F.: Standardization in platform stabilometry being a part of posturography. Agressologie *7:* 321–326 (1983).

Pyykkö, I.; Toppila, E.; Starck, J.; Aalto, H.: Computerized posturography: development of simulation and analysis methods; in Klaussen, Kirtane, Vertigo, nausea, tinnitus and hearing loss in cardio-vascular diseases, pp. 353–362 (Elsevier, Amsterdam 1986).

Taguchi, K.; Iijima, M.; Suzuki, T.: Computer calculation of movement of body's center of gravity. Acta Otolaryngol (Stockh.) *85:* 420–425 (1978).

H. Aalto, MSc, Institute of Occupational Health, Laajaniityntie 1,
SF-01620 Vantaa (Finland)

Adv. Oto-Rhino-Laryng., vol. 42, pp. 55–58 (Karger, Basel 1988)

Computer Analysis of Nystagmus Using a Syntactic Pattern Recognition

M. Juhola[a], *I. Pyykkö*[b]

[a]Department of Computer Science, University of Turku, Turku;
[b]Department of Otorhinolaryngology, University Central Hospital of Helsinki, Helsinki, Finland

Introduction

Determination of nystagmus from digitized eye movement signals has usually been performed by computing a velocity profile of the position signal and by examining this velocity [1]. We introduce an abstraction of the nystagmus signal which utilizes syntactic pattern recognition. The method is derived from an earlier work on saccades [2].

Preprocessing of the Nystagmus Signal

Eye movements are first recorded electro-oculographically with a sampling frequency of 400 Hz. A signal is filtered by a low-pass filter with a cutoff frequency of 70 Hz. The signal is then divided into consecutive segments. The length of each segment is 20 ms, covering 9 samples. For each segment, the velocity is computed by the method of least squares. If the velocity of a segment is nonnegative, this segment is transformed into symbol a; if it is negative, the segment is transformed into b. The signal is now a sequence of symbols a and b. Because fast phases of nystagmus last 30 ms or more [1], the shortest fast phases, having at least two segments, can be detected.

Syntactic Recognition of Nystagmus

Let us consider a signal in figure 1 of two nystagmus movements transformed as described above. The first slow phase is a sequence of symbols

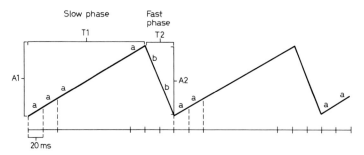

Fig. 1. An ideal nystagmus and its formal representation with symbols a and b.

a, and the fast phase a sequence of symbols b. We now present a formal language to abstract the nystagmus signal. Symbols a and b are so-called terminals. S', S, A, B, C, and D are the nonterminals. Productions are used to derive sequences of terminals. The first production is always:

(0) S' -> S,

in which S' is the start symbol. The derivation of a sequence is then continued with productions:

(1) S -> aaA
(2) A -> aA,

which produce, e.g. the first slow phase in figure 1. This is obtained by productions (0), (1), and repeatedly using (2) as follows:

$$S' => S => aaA => aaaA => \ldots => a^mA.$$

Thereafter, we apply productions:

(3) A -> bbB
(4) B -> bB,

which produce the first fast phase as follows:

$$a^mA => a^mbbB => a^mbbbB => \ldots => a^mb^nB.$$

Finally, production:

(5) B -> aa

is applied to obtain

$$a^mb^nB => a^mb^na^2,$$

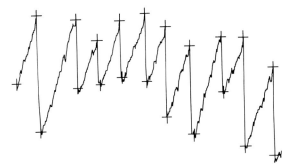

Fig. 2. Caloric nystagmus of 5 s.

which means that the end of the fast phase as well as the beginning of the subsequent movement have been found. The next movement is then represented in the same way.

If the nystagmus movement is in the opposite direction, we use productions

    S -> bbC
    C -> bC
    C -> aaD
    D -> aD
    D -> bb,

respectively. Each nystagmus movement is, as a terminal sequence of $a^m b^n$, a sentence of this formal language. Such sentences can be found from the transformed signal by using a program, namely parser. Terminal sequences are fed into the parser which derives these sequences applying the productions. The analysis program of nystagmus then recognizes fast and slow phases, minima and maxima.

Signals are sometimes quite uneven, even after filtering, due to noise and artifacts. Thus, we add productions:

    A -> baA
    D -> baD

to represent a possible short negative deflection in the positive velocity. The other way round, a single symbol a between symbols b is obtained by:

    B -> abB
    C -> abC.

An Experiment of the Method

Caloric nystagmus of a subject was recorded and preprocessed as mentioned above. A part of 5 s is shown in figure 2. This signal was contaminated by EMG noise. Maxima and minima, detected by the program, are shown by crosses. The recognition program was implemented in the Pascal of an HP 200 microcomputer.

References

1   Sills, A.W.; Honrubia, V.; Kumley, W.E.: Algorithm for the multiparameter analysis of nystagmus using a digital computer. Aviat. Space environ. Med. *46:* 934–942 (1975).
2   Juhola, M.: A syntactic method for analysis of saccadic eye movements. Pattern Recogn. *19:* 353–359 (1986).

M. Juhola, PhD, Department of Computer Science, University of Turku,
SF-20500 Turku (Finland)

Adv. Oto-Rhino-Laryng., vol. 42, pp. 59–64 (Karger, Basel 1988)

Modulation of Microphonics:
A New Method to Study the Vestibular System

H.P. Wit, B.J. Tideman, J.M. Segenhout

Department of Experimental Otolaryngology, University Hospital,
Groningen, The Netherlands

Introduction

Although its origin is still not fully understood, cochlear microphonics (CM) are widely used to study the hearing organ in various species. The disadvantage of the use of such a gross potential is that it does not give detailed information, for instance like recordings from neural fibers. On the other hand, the fact that microphonics provide an integrated view of (part of) the organ is sometimes advantageous.

Natural stimuli for the vestibular system have very low frequencies (below 10 Hz). This may be the reason that, due to technical difficulties, microphonics have not been used to study it.

However, the vestibular system is also sensitive to frequencies in the audio range [Tullio, 1929; Mikaelian, 1964; Young et al., 1977; Wit et al., 1984], and we have recently shown that audio-frequency stimuli can evoke a microphonic response from the vestibular system of pigeons [Wit et al., 1986].

In this paper we present results from measurements in which vestibular microphonics are used as a tool to study the response of the vestibular system to rotational stimuli in the natural frequency range.

Material and Methods

Experiments were performed in 34 homing pigeons (*Columba livia*), from which the membraneous cochleas were removed more than 4 weeks prior to an experiment. This operation slightly affects the vestibular system, as we learned from experiments performed too soon after cochlea extirpation; but within 4 weeks complete recovery takes

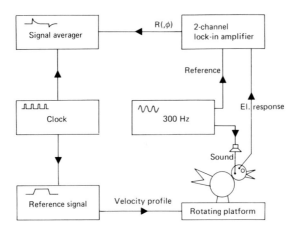

Fig. 1. Schematic of stimulation and recording equipment. The clock synchronizes signal averager and reference signal generator. The lock-in amplifier is used in the magnitude-phase mode.

place. The bird was placed on an electronically controlled rotating platform with its lateral canals in a horizontal plane and anesthetized with halothane (1%) in oxygen (1 liter/min). A 300-Hz constant amplitude pure tone (70 dB SPL) was delivered to the vestibular system through ear canal and columella, using a silastic tube. A small hole was cut in the bony wall of the lateral canal. This fenestration does not affect the membraneous part of the vestibular system, and by creating a 'round window' it makes the vestibular system more sensitive to sound. The vestibular microphonics potential, evoked by the pure tone stimulus, was measured with differential thin wire electrodes. One electrode contacted perilymph through a small hole in the top of the horizontal ampulla; the other was placed in a hole in the vestibulum. The amplitude of the microphonics potential was measured with a two-phase lock-in analyzer (EG&G 5206) and recorded with a signal averager (Datalab DL 4000) as shown in figure 1. The platform was rotated with a sinusoidal or trapezoidal velocity profile. As a rule responses to 8 full rotational cycles were averaged.

Results

A sinusoidal velocity profile for the rotating platform induces a sinusoidal modulation of the amplitude of the sound-evoked microphonics potential for low velocity (and acceleration) values (fig. 2, upper trace). With a stronger rotational stimulus distortion of the microphonics envelope occurs (fig. 2, lower trace).

A trapezoidal velocity profile creates sudden changes in microphonics amplitude, followed by an exponential decay. For high acceleration values a

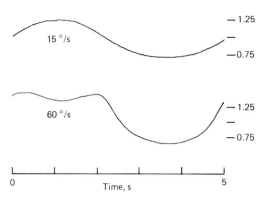

Fig. 2. Magnitude of microphonics potential on a relative scale during 1 cycle (0.2 Hz) of sinusoidal rotation of pigeon. Maximum acceleration during registration of the lower graph was 75 °/s².

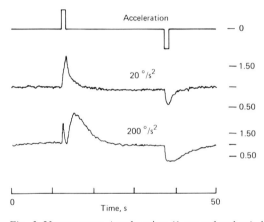

Fig. 3. Upper trace: Acceleration (1-second pulses) during 1 rotational cycle with trapezoidal velocity profile. Middle and lower trace: Magnitude of microphonics potential. Polarity of microphonics changes is in accordance with Ewald's second law.

sharp extra minimum, coinciding with offset of the acceleration pulse, appears in the response envelope (fig. 3).

The above results can successfully be described with a model. To illustrate this figure 4 gives a computerfit to a recorded microphonics envelope. Such model fits to the decaying microphonics envelope after an acceleration pulse (fig. 3) yield different decay time constants for different

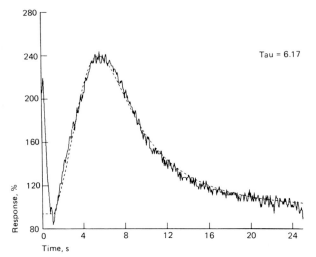

Fig. 4. Least-squares computerfit (dotted line) to microphonics potential (solid line) after offset of acceleration pulse (at t = 1 s).

acceleration values. In first approximation the relation between time constant τ (s) and acceleration a ($°/s^2$) can be given by:

$$\tau = 1.88 \ln a - 3.64 \ (20 \leqslant a \leqslant 300).$$

Discussion

The observed microphonics potential modulation during and after rotational acceleration can be described with a model that assumes a sigmoid-shaped relation between hair cell conductance and hair bundle deviation [Hudspeth and Corey, 1977]. It is further assumed that the 300-Hz pure tone stimulus causes a small amplitude oscillation of the hair bundle (with magnitude $\Delta\varphi$), leading to conductance variations $\Delta\sigma$ (fig. 5). Another assumption is that the measured microphonics potential is proportional to these conductance variations. This leads to a relation between microphonics amplitude and low frequency hair bundle deviation with a peaked shape, as given in the lower part of figure 5. If strong rotational stimuli deviate the hair bundles on the crista beyond the value φ_0, a decrease of microphonics amplitude occurs. This explains the shape of the lower graphs in figures 2 and 3.

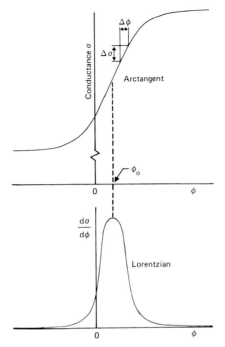

Fig. 5. Upper graph: Assumed relation between hair cell conductance and hair bundle deviation angle. Lower graph: First derivative of upper graph, giving relation between microphonics potential and hair bundle deviation for 'average' hair cell.

Figure 4 shows that also quantitatively the model does describe the obtained results very well. The further assumption that was made to fit the data in this figure was that starting right after offset of the acceleration pulse (at t= 1 s) the 'average' hair bundle returns to its zero position in an exponential way ($\varphi[t] = \varphi_{max} \cdot \exp[-t/\tau]$). Time constants τ for this return depend on the strength of the preceding stimulus. For relatively weak acceleration pulses (20 °/s²) τ is approximately 2 s; for strong pulses (300 °/s²) τ increases to a value of 7 s. A possible explanation for this phenomenon (observed in all pigeons under study) is that weak acceleration pulses stimulate a restricted area of the crista, where only short time constant hair cells are present; while with stronger stimuli a larger area of the crista is involved (where also long time constant hair cells are present). A place dependency for neurally recorded (hair cell?) time constants was demonstrated by Suzuki et al. [1986] for the crista of the hortizontal canal of the bullfrog.

A serious consequence of the above speculations is that the classical torsion pendulum model cannot adequately describe the functioning of the semicircular canal system on a single (neural) unit scale. A thorough discussion of this problem has recently been given by Lewis et al. [1985].

References

Hudspeth, A.J.; Corey, D.P.: Sensitivity, polarity, and conductance change in the response of vertebrate hair cells to controlled mechanical stimuli. Proc. natn. Acad. Sci. USA *74:* 2407–2411 (1977).

Lewis, E.R.; Leverenz, E.L.; Bialek, W.S.: The vertebrate inner ear, pp. 181–186 (CRC Press, Boca Raton 1985).

Mikaelian, D.: Vestibular response to sound: single unit recording from the vestibular nerve in fenestrated deaf mice (Df/Df). Acta oto-lar. *58:* 409–422 (1964).

Suzuki, M.; Harada, Y.; Sato, S.: An experimental study on the isolated lateral semicircular canal of the bullfrog. Archs Oto-Rhino-Lar. *234:* 27–30 (1986).

Tullio, P.: Das Ohr und die Entstehung von Sprache und Schrift (Urban & Schwarzenberg, Berlin 1929).

Wit, H.P.; Bleeker, J.D.; Mulder, H.H.: Responses of pigeon vestibular nerve fibers to sound and vibration with audiofrequencies. J. acoust. Soc. Am. *75:* 202–208 (1984).

Wit, H.P.; Kahmann, H.F.; Segenhout, J.M.: Vestibular microphonic potentials in pigeons. Archs Oto-Rhino-Lar. *243:* 146–150 (1986).

Young, E.D.; Fernandez, C.; Goldberg, J.M.: Responses of squirrel monkey vestibular neurons to audio-frequency sound and head vibration. Acta oto-lar. *84:* 352–360 (1977).

H.P. Wit, ENT Department, University Hospital,
P. O. Box 30.001, NL-9700 RB Groningen (The Netherlands)

Adv. Oto-Rhino-Laryng., vol. 42, pp. 65–71 (Karger, Basel 1988)

Statistical Identification of the Extent of a Peripheral Vestibular Deficit Using Vestibulo-Spinal Reflex Responses[1]

J.H.J. Allum, E.A. Keshner, F. Honegger, C.R. Pfaltz

Division of Experimental Audiology and Neurootology, Department of ORL, University Hospital, Basel, Switzerland

One of the aims of our research on human postural control has been to identify those vestibulo-spinal EMG responses and biomechanical measurements that best define a patient as belonging to a particular clinical population. Specifically the ENT specialist would wish to know if a patient can be classified as a normal, a patient with a unilateral peripheral vestibular deficit, or a patient with a bilateral deficit. The Romberg test, which is normally employed for this purpose, is not sensitive to vestibular dysfunction [2, 4], probably because only spontaneous sway movements on a fixed support surface can be analysed. Recent work studying the postural control of patients on a moving support surface has suggested, however, that the size of reflex responses induced by rotating the surface about the ankle joint are related to the clinically defined vestibular deficit [2, 3]. Here though, a statistical technique which could be used to classify each person tested into a specific patient population was not developed. Assuming such a technique was available it would be useful to know if it could depend on simple-to-measure biomechanical measurements such as ankle torque or body sway to classify patients or whether more complicated measurements such as surface EMG recordings were also required.

With the goal of developing a classification technique in mind, a stepwise discriminant analysis (BMDP 7M) was performed on the sway stabilising responses of 10 normals, 15 patients with unilateral peripheral vestibular deficit (UNILATS) tested twice, once at onset of their deficit and again 2

[1] The research was supported by Grant 3.148-0.85 from the Swiss National Research Fund.

months later when central compensation for the deficit was in progress, and 5 patients with bilateral deficit (BILATS). Postural reflexes were elicited by 10 consecutive 40 °/s ankle dorsiflexion rotations of the support surface on which the subject stood.

The methods and measurement techniques employed in this study duplicate those described elsewhere [3]. Essentially surface EMG signals were recorded from 3 muscles; tibialis anterior (TA), soleus (SOL) and from the upper fibres of trapezius covering neck extensor muscles (TRAP). Biomechanical recordings included torque about the ankle joint measured with a strain gauge system, and head and body accelerations recorded using angular acceleration transducers mounted respectively on a helmet and a breast plate harnessed to the chest.

For the first and main step in the analysis, areas of EMG responses in the SOL, TA and TRAP muscles as well as measurements of ankle torque were employed. These were divided into a number of 40 and 80 ms intervals as shown in figure 1 where responses of a normal subject are shown. The intervals consisted of two short latency periods, 40–80 and 80–120 ms after rotation onset, a medium latency (ML, 120–200 ms) and a long latency (LL, 200–280 ms) interval for a total of 16 variables. For ankle torque measurements these intervals were delayed 25 ms to account for the electro-mechanical coupling delay between the appearance of EMG activity and contraction force in a muscle. Analyses were run for two test conditions: (1) eyes open with means of the first 3 and second 7 trials (thus accounting for adaptation effects [3]); (2) eyes closed with means of the first 3 and second 7 trials. Adaptation ratios were also included in the analysis since adaptation, the amount by which EMG responses in the ankle muscles decrease with successive trials, has been claimed to be a variable capable of separating normals from vestibular deficit patients [2]. The adaptation ratio was defined for all ML and LL EMG and torque responses as the quotient of the average for the second 7 to first 3 trials. As a second step in the analysis, response latencies were included with no improvement in the classification procedure. Finally, the frequency, phase and amplitude of the head and body angular accelerations were entered into the analysis.

The stepwise discriminant analysis generates two outputs that help classify a subject as normal or not. Firstly the variables that should be used to classify a subject as belonging to one or the other population are identified in order of their significance. Secondly, the linear combination of these variables, i.e. the discriminant function or classification vector, that indicates the separation of the populations is established. When attempting to separate

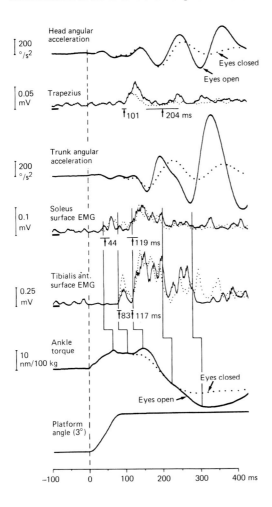

Fig. 1. Averaged responses of the first 3 trials to ankle dorsiflexing rotations of a 31-year-old normal standing with eyes open (solid line) and eyes closed (dotted line). The null level for EMG activity is marked with a short horizontal bar at the beginning of the EMG traces. The zero latency reference is given by a vertical dashed line, and corresponds to the first inflexion of platform velocity. Average values of EMG burst onset latencies are marked by a vertical arrow. A horizontal bar above the arrow indicates one standard deviation for that latency. An upward deflection of the head and trunk acceleration traces indicates backwards pitching angular acceleration. Increasing plantar flexion force on the support surface is represented by an upward deflection of the ankle torque curve. The intervals used to measure the area under an EMG response are shown by vertical thin lines on soleus and tibialis anterior EMG traces. These intervals are delayed 25 ms and then continued across the ankle torque trace to indicate torque measurement intervals.

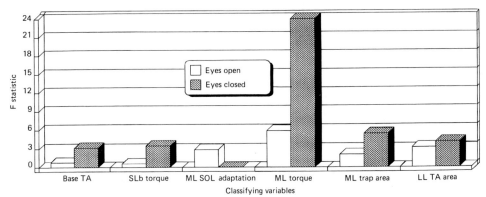

Fig. 2. Histogram of classification variables selected by the stepwise discriminant analysis to optimally separate normal and vestibularly deficient populations. The variable with the largest F value indicates the variable that best discriminates between the populations, the next largest F value, the next best variable and so on until a cut-off of $F = 2.6$ was reached.

more than two populations as here where four were present, more than one classification function may be required. For example, two populations may have nearly identical mean values for one measurement variable that can be used to separate them from a third population but significantly different means for another measurement variable. Figure 2 shows the specific variables that were most useful in distinguishing between the populations together with the F value for the variable prior to entering the discriminant analysis. High F values in the figure indicate the most significant variables. Once variables are entered on the basis of highest F value above a selected, fixed level (usually 2.6, equivalent to p < 0.1 for the number of DOF we used), the covariation of each entered variable is removed from the remaining variables before a new one-way analysis of variance and resulting F is determined for each remaining variable. For example, as shown in figure 2, ML torque is an important classifying variable under both eyes open and closed conditions, but neither TA nor SOL ML EMG area is specified, even though both are significantly smaller than normal in vestibular deficit patients [3]. Both TA and SOL ML EMG areas are highly correlated with ML torque and ML torque has a smaller variance. The selection of the same small subset of the variables for both eyes open and closed conditions (particularly ML torque, ML TRAP area and LL TA area) from among those entered, lends strength to their reliance as predictors of population parameters for our

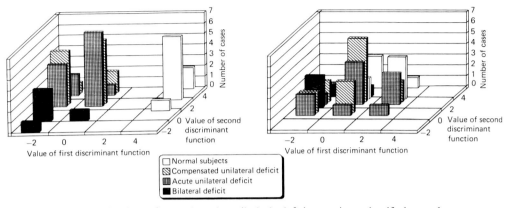

Fig. 3. Distributions of normals and vestibularly deficient patients classified according to the linear combination of variables optimally separating the four populations (the two discriminant functions along the axes). Analysis for eyes closed trials on the left, eyes open on the right.

experimental paradigm. Of all adaptation ratios exploited only that reported by Black et al. [3] for ML SOL area, proved to be of assistance as a predictor though, as figure 2 shows, only at an F level of 3 (barely $p < 0.05$).

The reliability of this applied statistical technique for differentiating between the populations can be determined from the distribution of the values of the discriminant functions for each subject along the classification vectors derived from the classifying variables. The percentage of overlap between the populations appears as an incorrect classification. Figure 3 presents these distributions for eyes open and closed conditions. The tightest clustering into three distinct populations (normals, UNILATS and BILATS) was achieved under eyes closed conditions (left part, fig. 3). For this condition the classification procedure was 100% correct in predicting the group membership of each subject from all three populations. Within the UNILAT population the classification of acute and compensated UNILATS was less correct, 3 of the 15 UNILATS patients (20%) were incorrectly classified as either acute or compensated when in fact the alternative was true. Our 2-month interval between test periods for the UNILATS was based on the average time required for the vestibulo-ocular reflex (VOR) gain to return to a normal value following a unilateral deficit [1]. Our underlying assumption was that vestibulo-spinal reflex amplitudes would also assume normal values 2 months after onset of a unilateral deficit. In contrast to this assumption the stepwise discriminant analysis performed on vestibulo-spinal reflex responses indicates that UNILATS examined 2 months after deficit onset have responses different from those of normals and their test results are not exactly distinguishable from those stemming from an examination at deficit onset. Thus, it appears that the time required for central compensation to adjust vestibulo-spinal reflexes to normal is much longer than the 2-month period required for the VOR.

The right part of figure 3 documents the difficulty in distinguishing vestibular deficit patients from normals when vision can be used to compensate for the vestibular system deficiency. Under eyes open conditions the overlap between populations shown in figure 3 precludes a satisfactory classification for all except the BILATS. Some improvement in the eyes open classification was obtained by including head and body acceleration data in the statistical analysis. The frequency of the oscillations in the angular acceleration traces shown in figure 1 is less in the vestibular deficit populations and coupling between trunk and head shows delayed phase characteristics [3]. The improvement obtained in the eyes open conditions with this additional information did not, however, approach the efficient classification obtained for eyes closed conditions without head and body acceleration information.

Using a controlled postural sway stabilisation task we have attempted to target functionally significant variables and experimental conditions that would make it possible for the clinician to identify a subject as a member of a clinical group. These variables in order of significance are the ML change in ankle torque (between 145 and 225 ms), the area under the ML neck flexor (TRAP) EMG response (between 120 and 200 ms) and the area under the LL tibialis anterior EMG response (between 200 and 280 ms). Subjects should be tested under eyes closed conditions to ensure an efficient identification of the vestibular deficit. In this research balance deficits in patients with only peripheral vestibular deficits were explored. It is clear that the diagnostic potential of tests which elicit vestibulo-spinal reflexes using a moving support surface need to be exploited by considering the differences in posture control between patients with central and peripheral vestibular deficits.

References

1   Allum, J.H.J.; Yamane, M.; Pfaltz, C.R.: Long-term modifications of vertical and horizontal vestibulo-ocular reflex dynamics in man. I. After acute unilateral peripheral vestibular paralysis. Acta oto-lar. *105:* 328–337 (1988).

2　Black, F.O.; Wall, C. III; Nashner, L.M.: Effects of visual and support surface orientation references upon postural control in vestibular deficient subjects. Acta oto-lar. *95:* 199–210 (1983).

3　Keshner, E.A.; Allum, J.H.J.; Pfaltz, C.R.: Postural coactivation and adaptation in the sway stabilizing responses of normals and patients with bilateral vestibular deficit. Exp. Brain Res. *69:* 77–92 (1987).

4　Wall, C.III; Black, F.O.: Postural stability and rotation tests: their effectiveness for screening dizzy patients. Acta oto-lar. *95:* 235–246 (1983).

Dr. J. Allum, Division of Experimental Audiology and Neurootology,
Department of ORL, University Hospital, CH-4031 Basel (Switzerland)

Adv. Oto-Rhino-Laryng., vol. 42, pp. 72–76 (Karger, Basel 1988)

Influence of Pressure Loading to the External Auditory Canal on Standing Posture in Normal and Pathological Subjects[1]

I. Watanabe, H. Ishida, J. Okubo, H. Nakamura

Department of Otolaryngology, Tokyo Medical and Dental University, Tokyo, Japan

The purpose of this study is to investigate the influence of the minimum pressure loading to the external auditory canal on the static body balance, and to try to find some clinical significance of this test in the field of otoneurology.

Method (fig. 1)

The subjects were asked to stand on a stabilograph (Anima Co.) with eyes covered or closed and with the feet in the Romberg position. During this time based on a DC output of left and right swaying, starting to increase the pressure load on the external auditory canal acted as a trigger to cumulatively add to the swaying ten times during 10 s. Pressure loading was performed with a special device. A tube was introduced into the external auditory canal, and an attached cuff was filled with air to seal the tube in place. In order to be able to judge the effects of both increasing and decreasing pressure at one recording, the stimulus of progressively increasing pressure was applied from 0 to 5 s and then decreased in the next 5 s. External atmospheric pressure was regarded as 0 mm H_2O, and the maximum pressure was set at 4 levels, namely ± 25, ± 50, ± 100, and ± 200 mm H_2O, in order to be able to detect the threshold of postural sway. Ten trials were performed at each pressure level and summated lateral body sways were recorded.

Figure 2 is an example of the recording pattern. This case was diagnosed as classical Ménière's disease, and showed marked fluctuation of hearing. The result of the pressure loading test proved to be negative in the right ear, but in the left ear, during the increasing pressure stimulus, a deviation toward the right was observed, and with decreasing pressure, the direction of deviation was changed in ± 100 mm H_2O and ± 200 H_2O pressure levels.

[1] This study was supported by a grant from the Ministry of Health and Welfare (1986) and also by a grant from the Ministry of Education (Topic Number 61870068).

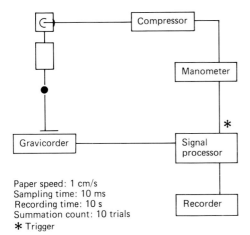

Paper speed: 1 cm/s
Sampling time: 10 ms
Recording time: 10 s
Summation count: 10 trials
∗ Trigger

Fig. 1. Block diagram of the pressure loading test.

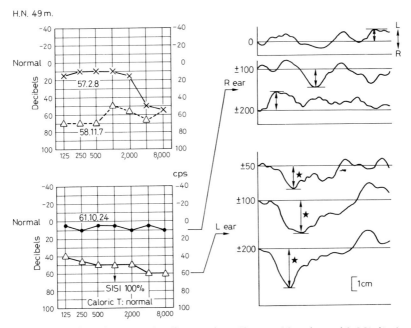

Fig. 2. Recording of pressure loading test in a 49-year-old patient with Ménière's disease. In this figure, the name of the era is expressed in Japanese style (SHOWA).

Table I. Results of pressure loading test in Ménière's disease, sudden deafness and normal subjects

	Positive	Negative	Total
Ménière's disease (n = 47)			
Group I			
Affected side	26 (62) *	16 (38)	42 (100)
Normal side	4 (22)	14 (78)	18 (100)
Group II			
Affected side	10 (45)	12 (55)	22 (100)
Normal side	4 (33)	8 (67)	12 (100)
Sudden deafness (n = 15)			
Affected side	3 (29)	12 (80)	15 (100)
Normal side	0	15 (100)	15 (100)
Normal subjects (n = 20)			
Right side	8 (40)	12 (60)	20 (100)
Left side	8 (40)	12 (60)	20 (100)

* p <0.01.

Subjects

Normal (Control) Group
The group of normal controls consisted of 20 healthy adults (8 males and 12 females, mean age 22.5 years) who underwent this test procedure.

Pathological Cases
Forty-seven cases of Ménière's disease and 15 cases of sudden deafness visited either Tokyo Medical and Dental University or the Municipal Komagome Hospital. The diagnoses were based on the diagnostic criteria of the Ménière's disease and Sudden Deafness Research Committee of the Ministry of Health and Welfare of Japan. The Ménière's disease group was subdivided into two groups according to the grade of fluctuation in the low-tone range of the audiograms. Cases which belong to group I showed fluctuation over 15 dB in the hearing level, and cases belonging to group II did not show clear fluctuations.

Results

The results were summarized in tables I and II. Eight out of 20 normal subjects showed positive responses. They usually appear symmetrically in both ears, except for one case, and the pressure needed to elicit positive

Table II. Asymmetric reaction to pressure loading test in Ménière's disease, sudden deafness and normal subjects

	Asymmetric	Symmetric	Total
Ménière's disease (n = 47)	26 (55)*	21 (45)	47 (100)
Group I	19 (63)	11 (37)	30 (100)
Group II	7 (41)	10 (59)	17 (100)
Sudden deafness (n = 15)	3 (20)*	12 (80)	15 (100)
Normal subjects (n = 20)	1 (5)*	19 (95)	20 (100)

*p <0.01

response was ± 100 mm H_2O or more. We thought that these were physiological responses.

In contrast, in pathological cases, especially in cases of group I Ménière's disease, the positive response usually appeared on the affected ear, and the response occurred even at a pressure level as low as ± 25 mm H_2O. We thought that these asymmetrical and very sensitive responses might be pathological. Statistically, the positive rate in the affected side of group I Ménière's disease was significantly higher in comparison with the positive rate of every other group.

Figure 3 shows the relationship between the loading pressure of minimum positive response (threshold of positive response) and the grade of the mean hearing level in the low-tone range in cases of Ménière's disease. Here, significant negative correlation between the hearing level and the minimum loading pressure level was observed and it was statistically significant. Further, not only the hearing level, but also the grade of fluctuation in the low-tone range in Ménière's disease showed a significant correlation with the positive response rate of pressure loading to the external auditory canal. On the other hand, we could not find a correlation between the positive rate and the results of glycerol tests or results of caloric tests.

From these findings, we considered that some kind of pathological process inside the labyrinth, which might be characteristic in Ménière's disease, exists in connection with the positive, pathological response to the pressure loading.

The pseudofistula sign in Ménière's disease is investigated by several authors [Nadol, 1974; Black, 1985; Watanabe et al., 1986]. However, we think that the fundamental knowledge is still lacking. Accordingly, in order

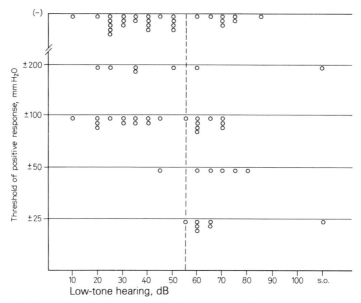

Fig. 3. Relationship between the loading pressure of minimum positive response and the grade of the mean hearing level in the low-tone range in cases of Ménière disease. o = earch ear; (–) = negative response (up to ±200 mm H$_2$O pressure loading).

to find the clinical significance of the pressure loading test, further study will be necessary.

References

Black, F.O.; Lilly, D.J.; Nashner, L.M.: Quantitative diagnostic test for perilymph fistula. Am. J. Otol. suppl., p. 39 (1985).

Nadol, J.B., Jr.: Positive Hennebert's sign in Ménière's disease. Archs Otolaryngol. *100:* 273–278 (1974).

Watanabe, I.; Ishida, H.; Okubo, J.; Niizeki, Y.: Influence of pressure loading to the external auditory canal on the stepping movement and standing posture. Jap. J. hum. Posture *6:* 93–100 (1986).

Isamu Watanabe, MD, Department of Otolaryngology, Tokyo Medical and Dental University, 5-45, 1-chome Yushima, Bunkyo-ku, Tokyo 113 (Japan)

Adv. Oto-Rhino-Laryng., vol. 42., pp. 77–80 (Karger, Basel 1988)

A Computer-Based Consultation System (Expert System) for the Classification and Diagnosis of Dizziness[1]

E. Mira[a], *R. Schmid*[b], *P. Zanocco*[a], *A. Buizza*[b], *G. Magenes*[b], *M. Manfrin*[a]

[a]Otorhinolaryngological Clinic and [b]Department of Computer and Systems Science, University of Pavia, Pavia, Italy

Expert systems (ES), or knowledge-based systems, are a new tool for information processing developed by the branch of computer science known as artificial intelligence. They are aimed to help professionals to solve problems in a given domain of the human knowledge (for instance medical diagnosis, chemical analysis, etc.), by making available the knowledge and the expertise of specialists in that domain. They are characterized by the capability of managing and processing large amounts of knowledge. This feature enables them to emulate the behaviour of a specialist when taking a decision.

ES consist of (1) a set of algorithms (inference engine) which represent the method of reasoning, (2) a 'knowledge base' which contains the body of facts, statements, and deductive rules peculiar to the domain of application, and (3) a set of data which contains the available information about the case or situation to be analysed. The inference engine applies the knowledge base to the data in order to infer conclusions, i.e. interpretations, diagnoses, suggestions, validation of hypotheses, etc.

A specific characteristic of ES is their ability to justify their own conclusions by making the underlying reasoning explicit. This feature definitely differentiates ES from more traditional computerised diagnostic aids (such as the decision trees), and greatly enhances their level of interactivity. Thanks to this possibility, ES can also be proposed as powerful tools for education. At present, medicine is the discipline were the largest number of ES has been developed. Existing applications concern either diagnosis or

[1] Work supported by CNR and HUSPI Project.

therapy in many different medical fields. All these applications are still limited, and no ES has yet become a routinary clinical tool. However, they already display interesting performance and remarkable reliability [1, 2].

Two years ago we started developing an ES (VERTIGO) for the classification and the diagnosis of different types of dizziness. VERTIGO is mainly conceived as (1) an educational tool for medical students and ENT residents, and (2) a diagnostic help for non-expert physicians such as general practitioners. Its goal is the classification of dizziness due to vestibular disorders and not a complete neurological diagnosis. Furthermore, we restricted the input data to VERTIGO to information derived from patient history only. One of the reasons for this choice is to stress the importance of this phase of the diagnosis procedure, which is often underestimated and neglected in favour of more complicated and expensive instrumental tests.

As a consequence of the above restriction, in VERTIGO attention has been mainly paid to the differential diagnosis of dizziness due to peripheral vestibular disorders, where a quite accurate and reasonably definite diagnosis can often be based on medical history only. VERTIGO has been developed by using the shell EXPERT [3], a package that helps constructing ES and has already been used to build a number of clinical consultation aids. An ES based on this shell contains HYPOTHESES, FINDINGS and RULES. The Hypotheses can be organised in a taxonomy and are the (diagnostic) conclusions that can be reached by the system. The Findings are the patient data. The Rules infer conclusions from the set of the available data, and thus represent the knowledge base of the system.

Table I gives the Hypotheses considered by VERTIGO, that is the different forms of dizziness it can classify, and their taxonomy. They are clustered in two groups: 'Vertigo' and 'Dizziness'. The former contains disorders having true vertigo as a major symptom, the latter disorders characterised by a non-specific, but still vestibular in origin, dizziness. Only its subset 'Non-Vestibular Dizziness' contains forms due to ophthalmological or mental, rather than vestibular, troubles. These forms, once identified, are not submitted to further investigation. In turn, the set 'Vertigo' contains two subsets: 'Paroxysmal Vertigo' and 'Vertigo due to Sudden Loss of Vestibular Function' (SLVF). In both, forms of vertigo different in aetiology are clustered according to their common pattern. The remaining forms of vertigo display more specific patterns. Consequently they are not clustered.

Patient history data are collected through a computer-controlled questionnaire. The sequence of questions is modified on line in order to adapt the

Table I.

Vertigo
    *Paroxysmal Vertigo
        **Benign Paroxysmal Vertigo of Childhood
        **Benign Paroxysmal Positional Vertigo
        **Paroxysmal Vertigo due to Vascular Disorder
        **Orthostatic Vertigo
        **Cervical Vertigo
        **Hepileptic Vertigo
        **Paroxysmal Vertigo due to Perilymphatic Fistula
    *Sudden Loss of Vestibular Function (Severe Vertigo Attack)
        **Severe Vertigo Attack due to Vestibular Neuritis
        **Severe Vertigo Attack due to VIII c.n. Neuritis
        **Severe Vertigo Attack due to Vascular Disorder
        **Severe Vertigo Attack due to Herpes Zoster Oticus
        **Severe Vertigo Attack due to Temporal Bone Fracture
        **Severe Vertigo Attack due to Suppurative Labyrinthitis
    *Ménière's Disease Vertigo
    *Cogan's Syndrome Vertigo
    *Vertigo due to Vascular Disorder
    *Vertigo due to Possible CNS Troubles
    *Atypical Vertigo due to Cerebellopontine Angle Tumour
    *Atypical Vertigo due to Herpes Zoster Oticus
    *Atypical Vertigo due to Temporal Bone Trauma
Dizziness
    *Dizziness due to Serous Labyrinthitis
    *Dizziness due to Cerebellopontine Angle Tumour (VIII c.n. Neuroma)
    *Dizziness due to Vascular Disorder
    *Dizziness due to Ototoxic Drugs
    *Dizziness due to Ototoxic Chemicals
    *Dizziness due to Incomplete Vestibular Compensation after SLVF
    *Dizziness due to Old Aged Ménière's Disease
    *Dizziness due to Temporomandibular Joint Syndrome (Costen's Syn.)
    *Dizziness due to Possible CNS Troubles
    *Non-Vestibular Dizziness
        **Dizziness originating from Mental Troubles
        **Dizziness originating from Ophthalmological Troubles

---

*Taxonomy   **Hypotheses.

---

questioning strategy to the information already acquired. In this way the system tries to emulate the diagnostic approach of an expert physician.

After unspecific questions concerning age, sex, and patient's general conditions, the key question is asked whether the patient is really complaining of vertigo. A positive answer triggers a set of questions concerning the characteristics of the vertigo: age and way of appearance, time course, strength, presence of precipitating factors. A negative answer triggers a different set of questions concerning other forms of dizziness that could still be related to vestibular disorders. The questionnaire is completed with questions on the presence of predisposing conditions and associated symptoms. At present the questionnaire contains about 40 questions concerning about 90 findings. Depending on selection, no more than 15–25 questions are actually asked during a typical diagnostic session.

After completing the questionnaire, VERTIGO presents a summary of the available data and then its diagnostic conclusions. Several conclusions can be proposed with their degree of certainty represented either as a numerical score or as probable/possible/suspected. Then many options can be selected: explanation of system's reasoning, modification of findings to check whether and how the conclusions would be changed, creation of a data base, etc.

At present, the knowledge base of VERTIGO is made of about 350 inference rules of different complexity. Two versions of the system are available. One runs on VAX computers, the other on IBM PC. So far, the system has been tested with satisfactory results on more than 120 cases taken from everyday clinical practice. The future steps of the project will be: (1) accurate validation of the system with the help of specialists who did not collaborate to its construction, (2) use of data from physical examination and instrumental tests as further findings, (3) more detailed classification of dizziness due to CNS disorders.

References

1   De Lotto, I.; Stefanelli, M. (eds): Artificial intelligence in medicine (North-Holland, Amsterdam 1985).
2   Szolovits, P. (ed.): Artificial intelligence in medicine (Westview Press, Boulder 1982).
3   Weiss, S.; Kulikowski, C.: EXPERT: a system for developing consultation models (Rutgers University, Department of Computer Science, CBM-TR-95 1979).

Prof. E. Mira, Clinica Otorinolaringoiatrica, Università di Pavia,
I-27100 Pavia PV (Italy)

Adv. Oto-Rhino-Laryng., vol. 42, pp. 81–84 (Karger, Basel 1988)

Computer Simulation of Eye Movements for Teaching and Training in Ocular Motor Pathology

P.L.M. Huygen[1]

Department of Otorhinolaryngology, Academic Hospital, Nijmegen,
The Netherlands

Anyone not (yet) familiar with ocular motor pathology may have difficulty in understanding textbook descriptions of eye movements, illustrations showing eye movement recordings or recordings as such. Demonstration of patients with clearly defined abnormalities can be particularly revealing. Such patients, however, are seldom available in person or even recorded on film or videotape and, if so, a lot of film or video editing work has to be done by professionals to make things readily accessible and understandable. Even then, not any recorded case will be representative or clear enough for teaching purposes and not every 'classical' type of pathology will be available to a single clinic. As an alternative, we have developed a special tool for teaching and training eye movement diagnostics by adopting computer methods for simulation.

The computer is a simple Commodore 64 micro ('hobby') computer with no other peripherals than a video monitor. The software resides in a menu-driven 64 K user cartridge (2×32-kbyte EPROM plus 1×8-kbyte EPROM containing a program which controls the menu routines for the selection of programs). This software consists of a Basic extension and two programs, 'Album 1' and 'Album 2'. These Basic programs include the required machine code, among which is the code for the high-resolution screen used as a background for the video animations and for the picture of the iris which is

[1] I am indebted to L.J.M. Huygen for developing the software in machine code and to A.J.R. Huygen for the major part of the artistic design.

Table I. Simulation items of 'Album 1' and the keys (A–Y) used for selection

Nystagmus		ENG	
A	To the right	W	record
B	To the left	X	record
C	Downbeat		
D	Upbeat		
E	Torsional, counterclockwise		
F	Torsional, clockwise		
G	of 1st degree		
H	of 2nd degree		
I	of 3rd degree		
J	Bilateral gaze		
K	Physiological endpoint		
L	Rebound		
M	in Abduction		
N	Bruns type		
O	Congenital fixation		
P	Latent fixation		
Q	Pendular	Y	record
R	in Ocular bobbing		
S	See-saw		
T	in Ping-pong gaze		
V	in Synergistic divergence		

a 'moveable object block' or 'sprite' which can be positioned anywhere on the screen by specifying two coordinates. Besides this, the EPROM contain a program for visual (saccade, smooth pursuit, optokinetic) stimuli which can be displayed on a television monitor with a large screen (subject distance some 80 cm) and a 'help' program indicating the startup procedure.

Part 1 of 'An Album of Simulated Eye Movements' ('Album 1') is a program for nystagmus simulation and part 2 ('Album 2') contains simulations of smooth pursuit eye movements and saccades. If the free choice option is used, a menu appears. After the selection of any item from this menu, a title is first displayed and then the simulated clinical picture or the ENG/EOG-record, whereafter the menu returns. The simulation items are presented in tables I and II; they are systematically discussed in a syllabus text which also refers to the literature.

A training option is available for both part 1 and part 2. The simulation item is randomly selected without text (only the stimulus is mentioned if

Table II. Simulation items of 'Album 2' with selection keys

Smooth pursuit		EOG	
A	Normal	O	record
B	Defective to the left	P	record
C	Defective to both sides	Q	record
Saccades			
D	Normal	R	record
E	General slowing	S	record
F	Bilateral INO	T	record
G	Abducens dysfunction right	U	record
H	Overshoot	V	record
I	Voluntary nystagmus	W	record
J	Ocular flutter		
K	Macro square wave jerks		
L	Opsoclonus/opsochorea		
M	Hypermetria	X	record
N	Multiple-step hypometric	Y	record

essential) and the student has to indicate a tentative diagnosis from the menu by pressing the appropriate key. The computer then shows whether this diagnosis is or is not correct and updates a score.

This software became available for teaching and training purposes in the spring of 1986. It is used by residents and assistants (otorhinolaryngology, neurology, ophthalmology) for postgraduate education and for training laboratory technicians. In our curriculum for the specialization in otorhino-laryngology, presenting the syllabus with all available simulations, including the simultaneous slide projection of original ENG/EOG recordings and some preliminary training, takes about 2 h. In an interuniversitary postgraduate course on vestibular examination for ENT specialists, a similar presentation of the most important items takes about 1 h. Just a few items can be selected for presentation in courses for general practitioners to let them get 'a feeling for nystagmus'.

The simulations are also available on 2 video cassettes (PAL/U-matic or VHS) of 1 h each. The first 12–15 min is taken by the sequential display of all simulations (arranged according to the syllabus) and the last 45 min can be used for training; after each simulation the menu is displayed for 5 s with the text 'Your diagnosis should be...' and then the correct answer is shown for 3 s.

The general experience is that this type of video simulation and computer-assisted instruction makes learning the essentials of eye movement pathology much easier. It can make the study and training program more efficient and certainly not at the cost of pleasure. The 'video textbook' can be also used as a reference manual in case of doubt about the (clinical) observations.

P.L.M. Huygen, PhD, Department of Otorhinolaryngology, Academic Hospital, Philips van Leydenlaan 15, NL-6500 HB Nijmegen (The Netherlands)

Adv. Oto-Rhino-Laryng., vol. 42, pp. 85–89 (Karger, Basel 1988)

Superimposition of ENG Recording on Video Eye Movements (Congenital Nystagmus)

N.S. Longridge[a], *S.F.J. Pilley*[b]

[a]Division of Otolaryngology, [b]Department of Ophthalmology,
University of British Columbia, Vancouver, Canada

Introduction

The telefactor VIII is a video recorder which allows direct superimposition of an electronystagmography (ENG) signal onto a TV camera picture of the patient's eyes as they move (fig. 1). This equipment was acquired by the hospital electroencephalography department in order to record sleep EEG while observing the patient's activity related to rapid eye movement sleep and nocturnal seizures.

Use of a splitter inserter allows a portion of the screen to be given over to a second camera image. Drawbacks of this equipment designed for EEG biological signals are a short time constant and a cut-off to prevent overlap of signals. Up to 8 channels of biological signal can be recorded and shown on the screen.

Figure 2 demonstrates the equipment. The technique is useful for recording unusual eye movements with the resultant ENG pattern that occurs instantly visible at the time the eye movement happens. The position of the eye in relation to the target stimulus can be followed. This technique allows production of teaching tapes for ENG study of eye movement disorders.

As this is a Bárány Society meeting, we chose a disorder described by Bárány to demonstrate this technique. In 1921 Bárány [1] devoted a few lines of an article on optokinetic (OKN) or as he called it railroad nystagmus to reversal of this phenomenon in the presence of spontaneous nystagmus (congenital nystagmus, CN).

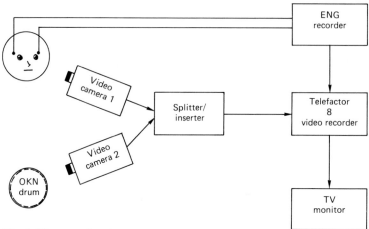

Fig. 1. Diagram of equipment.

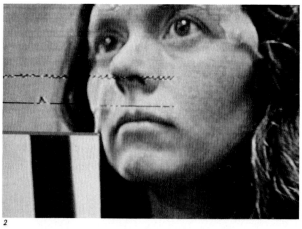

Fig. 2. Photograph taken from TV screen showing ENG superimposed on eye movements with stimulus observed in the left corner.

The standard texts often suggest that OKN reversal is pathognomonic [2–4] of CN and some have even suggested that absence of a pattern of reversal casts doubt on this diagnosis [2].

This is at variance with the usual clinical experience, it is frequently difficult to identify a pattern of OKN reversal in patients with most of the features of congenital nystagmus which are summarized in table I.

Table I. Characteristics of congenital nystagmus

Binocularity, eye movement the same in both eyes
Similar amplitude in each eye
Absence of oscillopsia
Uniplaner – usual horizontal nystagmus
Diminution and damping by convergence
Absence with eye closure
Additional latent nystagmus component
Frequent association of small angle strabismus

The stimulus for OKN is variable, from hand-held drum (as Bárány used) to projected stripes on a screen or wall to full surround curtains. Stripe width and speed also vary. Results between studies vary not surprisingly as the stimulus is not standardized.

In spite of the usual difficulty in demonstrating OKN reversal clinically in patients with CN, we did notice over a number of years that a reversal phenomenon was demonstrable in a few patients and that all of these patients had a very tight null zone or neutral zone. Furthermore, each of these patients when tested with the usual OKN drum tended to shift fixation to the leading edge of the drum. Consequently, we wondered whether the rare appearance of apparent OKN reversal was a manifestation of the appearance of an underlying gaze nystagmus where the OKN was suppressed and overidden by the gaze nystagmus.

Methods

The present video recording study was done using a hand-held 20-cm drum as per Bárány. It was held about 50 cm in front of the patient and rotated at about 100–150 °/s. The central 10° of the visual field is stimulated. The stripes are separated at 15° per pair (one black and one white).

A patient with clinically diagnosed congenital nystagmus showing evidence of apparent OKN reversal was identified. The clinical diagnosis was based on a long-standing history of nystagmus without oscillopsia, the presence of a latent component to nystagmus, binocular similarity of a horizontal nystagmus and the presence of a small angle strabismus.

Recordings are made in a variety of fixation and movement patterns as detailed below; these recordings will be shown in video display during paper presentation.

Fixating drum freely – drum static
Fixating drum freely – drum rotating to right
Fixating drum freely – drum rotating to left
Fixating right drum edge – drum rotating to right
Fixating left drum edge – drum rotating to right
Fixating right drum edge – drum rotating to left
Fixating left drum edge – drum rotating to left

Fixating right drum edge – drum rotating to left and right
Fixating left drum edge – drum rotating to right and left

A number of additional patients were recorded in a similar manner.

Results

During analysis of the recordings it was clear that the major component determining the pattern of nystagmus was the position of gaze; the direction of drum rotation was irrelevant in any eccentric gaze position. This pattern of findings was present for all patients tested.

Discussion

It appears that the OKN reversal apparent in patients with congenital nystagmus is due to the manifestation of an underlying gaze-evoked nystagmus. The presence or absence of OKN reversal in patients with congenital nystagmus is therefore primarily an indication of the extent of the null zone and the consequent propensity to develop a gaze-evoked nystagmus.

The presence of an OKN reversal is only seen clinically in those patients with a tight null zone and the absence of OKN reversal does not preclude the diagnosis. The patterns of apparent OKN reversal seen in our patients were similar to those described by Halmagyi et al. [3]. These authors made the tacit assumption that all of their patients were suffering from congenital nystagmus on the basis that all had OKN reversal to a greater or lesser degree. Many of their patients had other potential neurological disorders.

There may be differences in gaze induction with differing stimulus presentations. The surround curtain form is likely to be less gaze-inductive than the more usual drum presentation since the drum has a definite edge. There appears to be a tendency for gaze to drift towards the leading edge assuming the drum speed is not too high. Stimulus, size, frequency and speed may all affect induction of gaze drifts; this would appear to be confirmed in a number of patients reported by LeLeiver and Barber [2] in whom stimulus speed variation altered the appearance and direction of nystagmus in a number of individuals. The consensus explanation of the origin of this pattern of reversal now favours a concept of abolition of true OKN induction by induction of underlying gaze nystagmus although Yee et al. [4] record the existence of a rare true OKN reversal. Clearly this is a variant rather than the common pattern seen in most patients. Whether this gaze-evoked pattern is due to a true gaze drift, as appears to be the case in our patients, or due to a physiological shift of the null zone without true physical gaze shift is questioned.

From a practical standpoint, clinically there is a general consensus that OKN is difficult to demonstrate at all in most patients with congenital nystagmus. We consider that reversal is certainly not pathognomonic for congenital nystagmus and usually represents an expression of an underlying gaze nystagmus and that the OKN itself is relevant only in alteration of effective gaze position.

References

1   Bárány, R.: Zur Klinik und Theorie des Eisenbahnnystagmus. Acta oto-lar. *3:* 260–265 (1921).
2   LeLeiver, W.C.; Barber, H.O.: Observations on optokinetic nystagmus in patients with congenital nystagmus. Otolaryngol. Head Neck Surg. *89:* 100–116 (1981).
3   Halmagyi, G.M.; Gresty, M.A.; Leech, J.: Reversed optokinetic nystagmus (OKN): mechanism and clinical significance. Ann. Neurol. *7:* 429–435 (1980).
4   Yee, R.D.; Baloh, R.W.; Honrubia, V.: Study of congenital nystagmus: optokinetic nystagmus. Br. J. Ophthal. *64:* 926–932 (1980).

Dr. N.S. Longridge, Division of Otolaryngology, 4th Floor, Willow Pavilion, Vancouver General Hospital, Vancouver BC V5Z 1M9 (Canada)

Adv. Oto-Rhino-Laryng., vol. 42, pp. 90–94 (Karger, Basel 1988)

A New Method for Evaluating Autonomic Nervous Function in Patients with Equilibrium Disorders

K. Taguchi. M. Kikukawa, Y. Miyashita, O. Fukazawa,
H. Yokoyama, K. Wada

Department of Otolaryngology, Shinshu University School of Medicine,
Matsumoto, Japan

Almost all the patients with equilibrium disorders have some autonomic dysfunction. For example, the patient with Ménière's disease shows drastic symptoms of nausea, vomiting, pale face, cold sweating and bradycardia during the episode of vertiginous attack. However, the evaluation of autonomic nervous function would not be easy in the routine clinic. It has been claimed that the R-R interval on ECG involves estimation of autonomic nervous control in patients with diabetes mellitus [Wheeler and Watkins, 1973; Bennett et al., 1978; Clarke et al., 1979]. We applied the R-R interval on ECG for estimating the autonomic nervous function in patients with equilibrium disorders.

Materials and Methods

Subjects. Sixty normal adults, 30 patients with peripheral vestibular disorders, 30 with central nervous disorders and 10 with orthostatic dysregulation were studied.

Methods. Each subject lay quietly for 15 min, then stood up slowly (within 10 s) and remained motionless for 15 min, and lay again for 15 min. ECG was monitored and recorded on the paper, and simultaneously fed into an R-R interval processor to measure individual R-R intervals of continuous 100 heart beats and to calculate coefficient of variation of R-R intervals (CV_{R-R}) by the following formula:

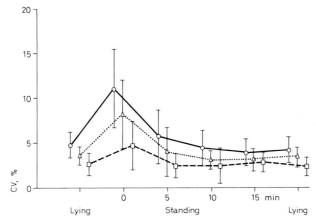

Fig. 1. CV_{R-R} curves of normal subjects. Mean ± standard deviation. Three age groups of normal subjects showed different time courses of CV_{R-R} with lying-standing-lying maneuver: 20- to 39-year-old (O); 40- to 59-year-old (△); 60- to 72-year-old (□).

$$CV_{R-R} = \frac{\text{Standard deviation of 100 R-R intervals}}{\text{Mean of 100 R-R intervals}} \times 100 \ (\%).$$

Results

Normal subjects were classified into 3 groups because of age differences, while CV_{R-R} curves showed a characteristic and consistent tendency through the 3 age groups. The CV_{R-R} was maximum at just after standing and then decreased to pre-standing value with some fluctuations (fig. 1).

Six different types of CV_{R-R} curves with the lying-standing-lying maneuver were obtained (fig. 2). There are close relationships between the types of CV_{R-R} curves and the autonomic nervous function: that is, type I to stable state, type II to parasympathetic dominance, type III to unstable autonomic nervous function, type IV to remarkably unstable autonomic nervous function, type V to relative sympathetic dominance and type VI to sympathetic dominance. Table I shows types of CV_{R-R} curves in normal subjects and patients with equilibrium disorders. There seems to be some relationship between causes or stages of equilibrium disorders and types of CV_{R-R} curves.

In some patients with autonomic imbalance the effect of autonomic agents was proved by the changes of type of CV_{R-R} curves (fig. 3).

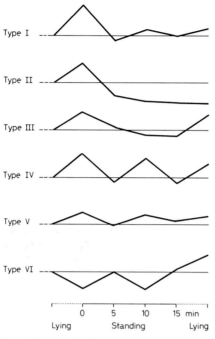

Fig. 2. Types of CV_{R-R} curves obtained from normal subjects and patients with equilibrium disorders.

Discussion

The heart-rate response is generated in the medulla oblongata and modified by intrinsic factors before the vagus nerve regulating beat-to-beat variation. Respiration is the most important intrinsic factor and its changes of depth and rate will alter the response. Parasympathetic and sympathetic perturbations are extrinsic factors, which affect the CV_{R-R} values. Standing would be a kind of sympathetic perturbation. Changing from lying to standing produces an integrated response of the cardiovascular system, which includes alterations in heart rate and blood pressure.

The present study deals with the clinical application of R-R intervals for evaluation of autonomic nervous function. A newly devised R-R interval processor can calculate the coefficient of variation and ratio of maximum to minimum of R-R intervals. We found a difference in the CV_{R-R} values

Table I. Types of CV_{R-R} curves in normals and patients with equilibrium disorders

Subjects	Types						Total
	I	II	III	IV	V	VI	
Normal	50	4	1	1	2	2	60
Peripheral vestibular disorders							
Intermittent stage	9	4	1			1	15
Active stage	1	11	2	1			15
Cerebral arteriosclerosis			7		1	2	10
Vertebulo-basilar artery insufficiency			1	5	1		7
Parkinsonism		1			4		5
Other central disorders	1	1	1		1	4	8
Orthostatic dysregulation	1	4	5				10
Total	62	25	18	7	9	9	130

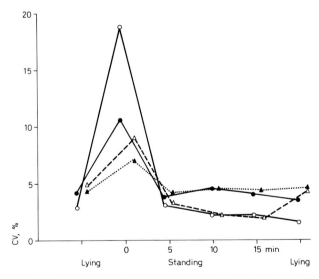

Fig. 3. Effect of autonomic agents: 52-year-old female with Ménière's disease, before (○) and after (●) administration of Bellergal; 40-year-old female with orthostatic dysregulation, before (△) and after (▲) administration of carnigen.

between normal subjects and patients with equilibrium disorders. The clinical value was also proved in the evaluation of the effect of autonomic agents. The results suggest the possibility of clinical application of the CV_{R-R} curve for autonomic nervous function tests.

References

Bennett, T.; Farquhar, I.K.; Hosking, D.I.; Hampton, J.R.: Assessment of methods for estimating autonomic nervous control of the heart in patients with diabetes mellitus. Diabetes *27:* 1167–1174 (1978).
Clark, B.F.; Ewing, D.J.; Campbell, I.W.: Diabetic autonomic neuropathy. Diabetologia *17:* 195–212 (1979).
Wheeler, T.; Watkins, P.J.: Cardiac denervation in diabetes. Br. med. J. *iv:* 584–586 (1973).

Kiichiro Taguchi, MD, Department of Otolaryngology, Shinshu University School of Medicine, 1-1 Asahi 3-Chome, Matsumoto 390 (Japan)

Adv. Oto-Rhino-Laryng., vol. 42, pp. 95–103 (Karger, Basel 1988)

Variations of Biphasic Head Shake Response: Physiology and Clinical Significance

John Spindler, Maurice Schiff [1]

Scripps Memorial Hospital, La Jolla, Calif., USA

Introduction

The head shake response is a provocational maneuver to evoke a decompensatory condition in patients with underlying vestibulopathy. While monophasic head shake responses reveal only the imbalance in the vestibular apparatus, biphasic head shake responses (BHSR) give additional information about the peripheral and central relationship. BHSR was first described by Vogel [1955] and became understood after Stenger's discovery of recovery nystagmus [Stenger, 1959]. Kamei [1975] first investigated BHSR in a systematic study. Sequentially alternating nystagmus beats in the first phase toward the sound ear (paretic nystagmus) and in the second phase toward the implicated ear (recovery nystagmus). We [Spindler and Schiff, 1982] reported the existence of a reversed response of BHSR, in which nystagmus beats toward the diseased ear in the first phase and toward the sound ear in the second phase. It became evident that a new classification of BHSR is needed to accommodate the different types of BHSR that appeared subsequently.

Materials and Methods

Two hundred and four ENG tracings of BHSR, obtained from patients with conventional DC oculography during a 5-year period, were selected. Patients were tested twice with the head shake maneuver; once with their eyes opened and once with their eyes

[1] The authors wish to express their gratitude to Prof. Stenger for allowing the reproduction of the figures and for his written information concerning the head shake response.

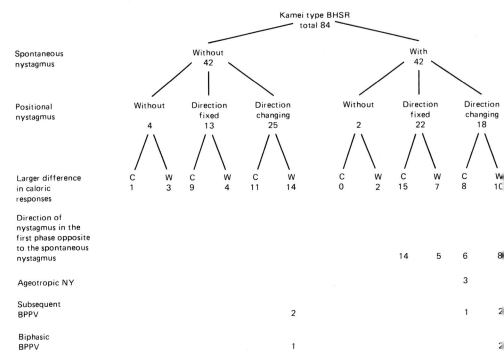

Fig. 1. Summary of ENG findings in patients with Kamei type BHSR. C=obtained with cold irrigations, W=obtained with warm irrigations.

closed. Movements of the eyes were observed through Frenzel glasses and were monitored simultaneously by ENG. With patients in a sitting position, spontaneous nystagmus was investigated in the same way as the head shake test. The types of BHSR were analyzed and related to ENG findings (caloric, difference in 30 and 44 °C responses, positional, and BPPV tests). Thirty-four patients were repeatedly tested, some of them were followed for many years.

Results

In the first group of 84 patients (fig. 1) with a classical Kamei type of BHSR, one half of the patients did not have recordable or observable spontaneous nystagmus, while the other half did have recordable, but not necessarily observable, nystagmus. Only 6 of 84 patients had no positional nystagmus. In patients with spontaneous nystagmus, 33 of 42 (78%) showed a change in direction of nystagmus; hence, in the first phase nystagmus beating toward the sound ear was opposite to the direction of spontaneous nystagmus. Ageotropic nystagmus was recorded in 3 patients. Subsequently, after the biphasic head shake response faded away, BPPV was observable in 5 patients, 3 of whom showed a *biphasic BPPV*.

A second group of 18 patients exhibited a pattern similar to the first group, but the nystagmus in the second phase was directed toward the calorically nonfunctional ear as determined by the ice-cold irrigation in Brünings position No. 5 (fig. 2). Spontaneous nystagmus in all patients of this group was beating toward the sound ear. A third group of 16 patients in whom the spontaneous nystagmus was beating toward the hypofunctional ear, as a result of irritation or central imbalance, showed an absence of the first phase and somewhat increased intensity of nystagmus beating toward the hypofunctional ear in the second phase. A fourth group consisted of 48 patients with a reversed BHSR response where the first phase nystagmus was beating toward the diseased ear. In 19 (67%) patients (fig. 3) the direction of nystagmus in the first phase was opposite to the direction of spontaneous nystagmus. Two more groups were examined: 8 patients with prolonged BHSR and 9 patients without any vestibular deficit with BHSR.

Discussion

Table I summarizes the types of BHSR and biphasic BVVP, since analogous processes may be involved. Reversed BHSR may have a peripheral or a central origin and both types show vestibular disorders. On the other hand, BHSR can be obtained as a single isolated finding in patients with central pathology without vestibular pathology.

In the first group BHSR as an isolated finding occurred only in 4 patients. In 33 patients the direction of nystagmus in the first phase became reversed from the direction of spontaneous nystagmus. This finding supports the concept of a preexisting recovery nystagmus beating toward the affected ear. Strong Kamei type responses in patients with recovered and symmetrical caloric function, as well as prolonged Kamei responses in patients with bilaterally diminished caloric function, indicate that the head shake test not only unmasks 'Nystagmus Bereitschaft' of the horizontal pair of canals, but also reveals pathology in other parts of the vestibular apparatus. Deficiencies, deceptive in partially compensated static equilibrium, are exposed only by a dynamic provocation with a head shake. The BHSR is the only test that

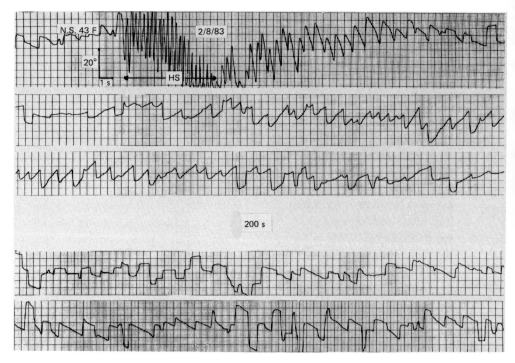

Fig. 2. Biphasic head shake response of a patient with an acoustic neuroma and left loss of function. Horizontal ENG derivation; upward deflection denotes right eye deviation. HS = Duration of head shake. First phase in the first row. Second phase starts in the second row and continues for 280 s when nystagmus reverts to right beating spontaneous nystagmus.

extrapolates status from the past and combines it with the present condition, so that the case history of the patient is recorded on a *compressed time scale.*

It is remarkable that the patients with incapacitating positioning vertigo (BPPV) remain unperturbed after a head shake test. In rare instances, however, BHSR may also occur as an intermediate stage toward complete recovery by way of BPPV. Three of 5 patients in the first group, who developed a subsequent BPPV, also showed a biphasic BPPV (fig. 4). Rotatory nystagmus, observable through Frenzel glasses, was seen to change its direction from beating toward the undermost ear in the first phase, to the uppermost ear in the second phase, when the patient maintained an unchanged head hanging position. We believe this to be a manifestation of recovery nystagmus analogous to the second phase in BHSR.

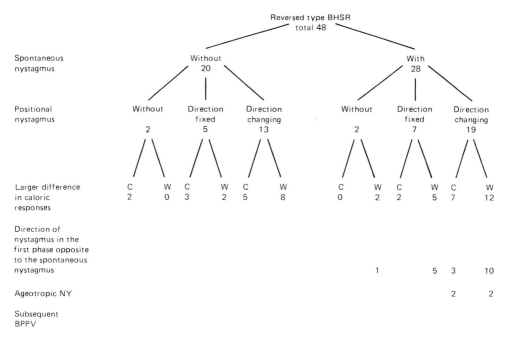

Fig. 3. Summary of ENG findings in patients with reversed type BHSR. C and W as in figure 1.

Patients in the second group with the second phase nystagmus beating toward the dead ear can neither be semantically nor prognostically considered the same as those in the first group whose function recovered despite similar ENG records of BHSR. For example, the BHSR in figure 2 was obtained from a patient who showed peripheral symptoms caused by a retro-labyrinthine pathology, namely a *left* acoustic neuroma. There is also a difference in the configuration of nystagmus; the recovery nystagmus is of smaller amplitude and not as intense. In the third group of patients who exhibited spontaneous nystagmus toward the implicated ear, the very absence of the first phase may be a significant finding.

Of the fourth group of 48 patients with reversed BHSR (fig. 5), 6 had Ménière's disease, 11 had had accidents, and 14 had a history of viral and infectious disease. The patients with Ménière's disease may provide some clues about the origin of the first phase BHSR. One patient showed low tone fluctuating hearing loss. Attacks of vertigo occurred 3 or 4 times a year. The reversed BHSR could be evoked before or after the attack and it did not

Table I. Interpretation of biphasic provocational responses

Condition and type	1st phase nystagmus toward	2nd phase nystagmus toward
Recovered function Kamei	sound ear paretic nystagmus	affected ear recovery nystagmus
Loss of function SP NY toward the sound ear	sound ear paretic nystagmus	nonfunctional ear central nystagmus
Loss of function SP NY toward the affected ear	absent	affected ear
Reversed type peripheral origin	affected ear irritation nystagmus	sound ear paretic nystagmus
Reversed type central origin	affected ear ?	sound ear ?
Central type no vestibular deficiency	either ear ?	either ear ?
Biphasic BPPV	undermost ear rotatory, paretic?	uppermost ear rotatory, recovery?

change. The right beating nystagmus in the first phase of BHSR mimicked a response to a 44 °C irrigation that causes a depolarization at the receptor level. The first phase originated in the right ear and was a peripherally evoked irritational nystagmus, while the second phase was a consequence of stronger spontaneous discharge from the left end organ. While it is an open question whether the head shake mechanics cause changes at the receptor level, it is known that a diseased labyrinth can trigger a peripheral nystagmus in both directions [Vogel, 1955].

The group of 8 patients with prolonged responses (fig. 6), 5 with reversed BHSR, showed an intensity and duration of nystagmus in the first phase that is not compatible with cupular mechanics; its origin may be central. Prolonged responses of patients with bilaterally diminished caloric responses suggest the possibility that the head shake causes not only a decompensation, but also a disinhibition.

Follow-up examinations discriminate peripheral from central causes in patients with reversed BHSR. Peripheral vestibulopathy is transient, while central pathology remains longer. In 9 patients a central origin of nystagmus was ascribed to the patients without any vestibular deficit and with strong BHSR.

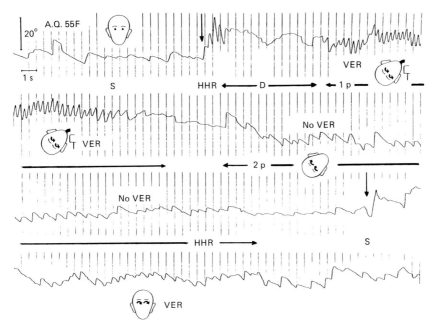

Fig. 4. Biphasic benign paroxysmal positional nystagmus (BPPV). ENG same as seen in figure 2. S = Sitting position; HHR = head hanging right position; D = delay in onset; 1p = first phase; rotatory nystagmus beating counterclockwise; 2p = second phase, clockwise nystagmus; VER = vertigo.

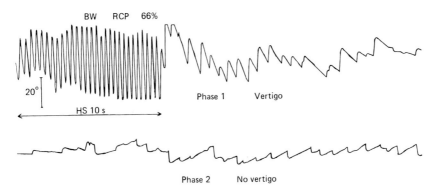

Fig. 5. Reversed biphasic head shake response, peripheral origin. Patient with Ménière's disease in the right ear. ENG same as in figure 2. RCP = Right canal paresis.

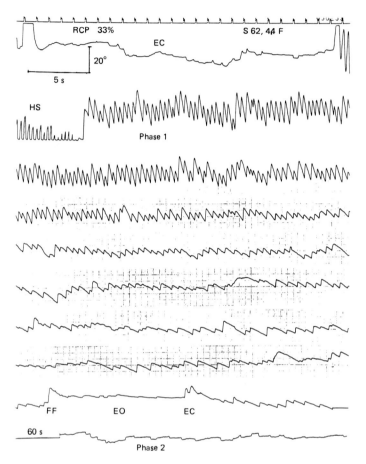

Fig. 6. Reversed biphasic head shake response, central origin. Prolonged first phase lasting over 200 s, ENG same as in figure 2. RCP = Right canal paresis; EO = eyes opened; FF = finger fixation; EC = eyes closed.

Conclusion

The push-pull phenomena between the central and peripheral nervous systems, revealed by BHSR, give information about the direction of nystagmus that is valuable in localizing the site of lesion.

References

Kamei, T.: Der biphasisch auftretende Kopfschüttelnystagmus. Arch. Oto-Rhino-Lar. *209:* 59–67 (1975).

Spindler, J.; Schiff, M.: A new type of head shake response and its significance. Report at Am. Neuroto. Soc., Palm Beach 1982.

Stenger, H.H.: 'Erholungsnystagmus' nach einseitigem Vestibularisausfall, ein dem Bechterew-Nystagmus verwandter Vorgang. Arch. Ohr.-Nas.-KehlkHeilk. *175:* 545–548 (1959).

Vogel, K.: Über klinische Anhaltspunkte zur Unterscheidung von peripher und zentral bedingtem Nystagmus. Dt. med. J. *6:* 53–58 (1955).

Dr. John Spindler, 13596 Freeport Road, San Diego CA 92129 (USA)

Adv. Oto-Rhino-Laryng., vol. 42, pp. 104–107 (Karger, Basel 1988)

A New Visual Suppression Test Using Postrotatory Nystagmus

Kazuhiro Teramoto, Eiji Sakata, Hidetaka Yamashita, Kyoko Ohtsu

Department of Neurotology, Saitama Medical School,
Saitama Irumagun, Moroyama, Japan

Introduction

The visual suppression test is a useful method for examining the function of visual fixation. But we often had trouble in examinations. Because caloric stimulation is such a strong stimulation, the patient having vertigo often vomits. If we consider the suffering and pain in patients, there is nothing better than a test which uses milder and easier stimulation.

Recently, we succeeded in a visual suppression test using a postrotatory nystagmus (fig. 1). We report here our new visual suppression test.

Method

The chair is accelerated at 0.3 °/s². The room is kept perfectly dark and the patient has closed eyes. The rotating velocity is increased until the maximum 90 °/s, and maintained at that level for 1 min. After that, the chair is suddenly stopped and the patient opens the eyes. After 5 s, we put the room light on and the patient fixates on the target for 5 s, then we put the room light off again to return perfect darkness. Eye movement is differentiated to obtain velocity measurements and clipped to display the slow-phase velocity (fig. 1).

Results

Normal Subjects. Figure 2 demonstrates a 22-year-old healthy woman. The left side of figure 2 shows the recording of the postrotatory method and the right side shows the one using the caloric method.

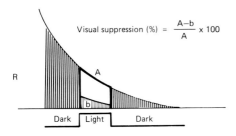

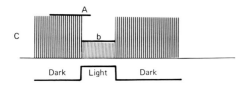

Fig. 1. Upper R shows recording of visual suppression test using postrotatory nystagmus. Lower C shows the use of a caloric method.

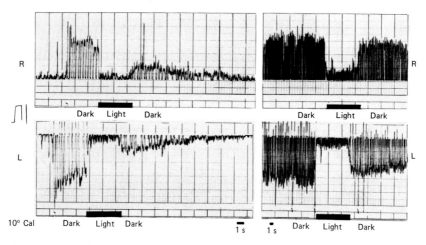

Fig. 2. A normal subject.

We performed the visual suppression test using the postrotatory nystagmus in 37 normal adults. The mean visual suppression ratio was $63 \pm 14\%$.

Cases with Failure of Fixation Suppression. Figure 3 demonstrates the case with failure of fixation suppression. Visual suppression of the slow-

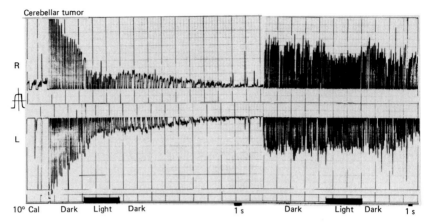

Fig. 3. Case of failure of fixation suppression with cerebellar tumor.

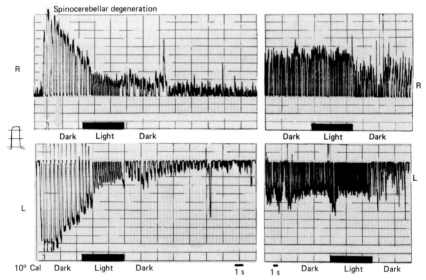

Fig. 4. Failure of fixation suppression with spinocerebellar degeneration.

phase velocity using postrotatory nystagmus was rotation to right 23.2%, rotation to left 5.6%, and the one using caloric stimulation was irrigation of right ear 12.4%, irrigation of left ear 0%.

Figure 4 demonstrates a visual suppression test in a patient with spinocerebellar degeneration. Visual suppression of the slow-phase velocity using postrotatory nystagmus was rotation to right 12.0%, rotation to left 15.6%, and the one using caloric stimulation was irrigation of the right ear 0%, irrigation of the left ear 17.4%.

Conclusion

This new method has various special advantages but, the most of all, it is milder than the one using caloric stimulation. Thus, it can be easily performed on aged men, children and a patient with motion sickness. Also, we get an almost perfect correlation with the caloric visual suppression test.

References

1   Takemori, S.; Cohen, B.: Visual suppression of vestibular nystagmus in rhesus monkeys. Brain Res. *72*: 203–212 (1974).

Kazuhiro Teramoto, MD, Department of Neurotology, Saitama Medical School, Saitama Irumagun, Moroyama 38, 350–04 (Japan)

Adv. Oto-Rhino-Laryng., vol. 42, pp. 108–115 (Karger, Basel 1988)

The Influence of Hyperventilation on Caloric and Optokinetic Responses in Normal and Pathological Subjects[1]

G.C. Modugno, S. Marcellini, A. Pirodda, E. Pirodda

Clinica Otorinolaringologica dell'Università di Bologna, Bologna, Italy

Hyperventilation has occasionally been found to be responsible for a more or less typical vestibular symptomatology [2, 5–7]. This observation has originated several studies aimed at assessing the characteristics of the phenomenon, identifying the mechanisms through which hyperventilation may influence the activity of the vestibular system, and evaluating whether and to what extent the phenomenon may be utilized for clinical purposes.

Hyperventilation has been known for a long time to induce a slowing down of the electrical activity of the cerebral cortex. A number of investigations have been carried out in order to obtain a better understanding of mechanisms through which hyperventilation influences the metabolism and the activity of different structures in the CNS. The most credited experimental evidence shows that reflex vasoconstriction, consequent hypoxia and the Bohr effect mediate this influence [3].

Furthermore, low CO_2 pressure may reasonably be thought to exert a depressing effect on the resting potential of neuron membranes, thus determining an increase in their excitability [1, 4].

Much less is known about the degree of sensitivity of different cortical and subcortical structures to oxygenation and metabolic changes induced by hyperventilation. It may be speculated that the cortex is among the most sensitive. A sustainable hypothesis, therefore, could be that hyperventilation influences the quantitative characteristics of vestibular reflex responses by depressing the activity of cortical structures involved in the efferent control of the vestibular function.

[1] The authors wish to thank Mr. Gino Mattei and Mr. Giuliano Morisi for their skilful technical support.

A more systematic investigation into the problem seems justified, not only on the basis of the intrinsic importance of a deeper understanding of mechanisms underlying such effects, but also in view of the possibility of a useful clinical application. Quantitative vestibulometry is classically limited in its clinical value by the discouraging individual and interindividual variability of measurements. Hyperventilation could find a place in improving the chances of being able to perform a reliable and meaningful quantitative analysis of vestibular reflex responses. The influence of hyperventilation on the behaviour of vestibular reflex responses may, on the other hand, be potentially of some help in the differential diagnosis of lesions affecting different sections of the vestibular system.

Materials and Methods

Ten normal persons (aged 25–33 years) served as test subjects. A monothermal caloric test (irrigation with 100 ml water at 44 °C in 30 s) and an optokinetic test (stare test) were utilized according to the usual standard procedures. Hyperventilation was applied for 2 min 30 s before and during the whole duration of the irrigation (30 s); for 3 min immediately before the optokinetic test.

Fourteen subjects suffering from different vestibular disturbances (6 cases among them due to pure central lesions), aged 16–66 years, average 42.5 years, were also examined with the optokinetic test. A velocity of 35 °/s was used. The test was administered and recordings were taken prior to and after 3 min of hyperventilation.

Quantitative parameters of nystagmus (frequency, amplitude of the slow and the rapid phase) were calculated by a computerized automatic analysis (processor 6502) based on an off-line interactive algorithm.

Average values of the mentioned parameters were calculated in normal subjects every 20 s for the caloric tests and every 10 s for the optokinetic test (total duration 40 s) and during the first 20 s following hyperventilation in the subjects suffering from vestibular lesions. Statistical significance of obtained data was calculated by means of a Wilcoxon signed rank test.

Results

Normal Subjects. ENG showed no *spontaneous* nystagmus either before or during hyperventilation.

Caloric Test. In comparison with reference 'normal' pre-hyperventilation values the frequency of nystagmic beats increased in a highly significant manner ($p < 0.01$) and the angular velocity of the slow phase in a clearly significant manner ($p < 0.05$) under the influence of hyperventilation (fig. 1).

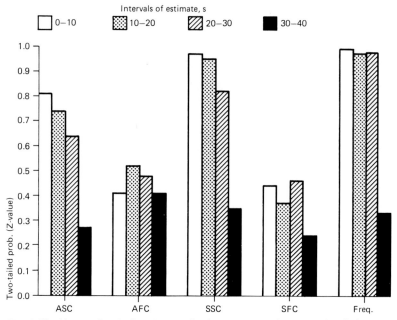

Fig. 1. Significance level of each quantitative parameter in a sample of 10 normal subjects during caloric test after hyperventilation. ASC=Amplitude of slow component; AFC=amplitude of fast component; SSC=speed of slow component; SFC=speed of fast component; Freq.=frequency.

Significance indexes were calculated on the pooled data from all tested subjects. The influence of hyperventilation on the quantitative parameters of the nystagmic reaction was observed to decrease gradually after the first 20 s following the end of hyperventilation.

Optokinetic Test. An increase in all of the quantitative parameters of the reaction, with the exception of frequency, was observed for all of the subjects. The statistical evaluation (carried out on the pooled data from all tested subjects) indicated a high significance ($p < 0.01$) of increase for all of the parameters (except frequency) during the first 10 s (fig. 2).

Pathological Subjects. A spontaneous nystagmus was present in 6 cases (4 among them showing a documented diagnosis of lesions in the CNS; one a suspected central lesion; one suffering from a vestibular neuritis). Spontaneous nystagmus when present was observed to increase under the influence

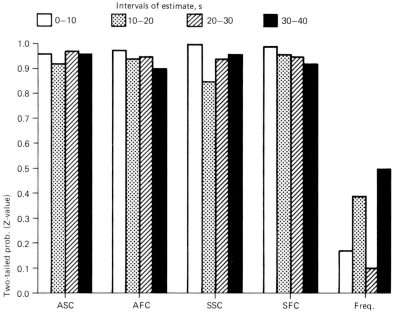

Fig. 2. Significance level of each quantitative parameter in a sample of 10 normal subjects during stare test after hyperventilation. Abbreviations as in figure 1.

of hyperventilation in all of its quantitative parameters in 5 cases. Spontaneous nystagmus disappeared during hyperventilation in one case (cerebellar lesion). In 2 patients a nystagmus appeared during hyperventilation (diffuse vascular disturbance with particular involvement of the cerebellum, one case; hyperventilation syndrome, one case).

Optokinetic Test. Of 8 cases showing spontaneous nystagmus before or during hyperventilation (table I, fig. 3), optokinetic stimulation evoked a homodirectional nystagmus, as compared to the spontaneous one, in 5 cases. All of the quantitative parameters showed decreased values during hyperventilation, as compared to the base values, in 2 patients (cerebellar lesion) out of 5. As for the other 3 cases (arachnoid cyst; hyperventilation syndrome; diagnosis undefined), the angular velocity of the slow component always remained unchanged, the angular velocity of the fast component decreased in 2 cases and remained unchanged in one, the frequency increased in 2 cases and remained unchanged in one (arachnoid cyst). The amplitude of the slow and the fast components always decreased. The direction of the optokinetic

Table I. Effect of hyperventilation on spontaneous nystagmus and on speed of slow component and frequency of optokinetic nystagmus in pathological subjects

Patient No.	Spontaneous nystagmus		Direction of OKN (as compared to spontaneous hystagmus	SSC	Frequency	Pathology
	before	during				
1	left	+++	contra	–	+	central
2	left	---	ipsi	--	–	central
3	left	+++	ipsi	--	–	central
4	right	+++	ipsi	*	*	central
5		left	contra	++	+++	central
6	right	+++	ipsi	*	+++	(central)
7	left	+++	contra	*	*	periph.
8		right	ipsi	*	++	(central)

SSC = Speed of slow component; * = unchanged; –/+ = <10%; --/++ = 10–20%; ---/ +++=>20%.

nystagmus was contralateral, as compared to the spontaneous one, in 3 patients. Under the influence of hyperventilation in 1 case (expansive paratentorial lesion) all of the parameters except frequency showed decreased values, in the second case (diffuse vascular lesions with particular cerebellar involvement) the frequency and the angular velocity of the slow phase increased while the other parameters decreased, in the third case (hyperventilation syndrome) the response remained substantially unchanged.

In 6 cases without spontaneous nystagmus (table II) an increase in the angular velocity of the slow phase was never observed. It decreased in 2 cases (central undetermined lesion; diagnosis uncertain), and remained unchanged in the other cases. The angular velocity of the fast component always remained substantially unchanged.

Discussion

The results of our investigations not only confirm previous observations about the influence of hyperventilation on the quantitative characteristics of the optokinetically induced nystagmus but show beyond any doubt that also the vestibulo-ocular reflex response produced by the thermic stimulation is

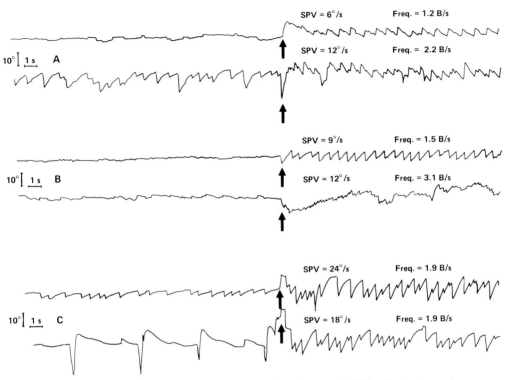

Fig. 3. Effect of hyperventilation before and after the start of OKR stimulus (arrow) in 3 patients with cerebellar lesions. Upper trace = Control test; lower trace = hyperventilation test; SPV = slow phase velocity; Freq. = frequency. *A, B* Induced nystagmus during hyperventilation and increased OKR nystagmus. *C* Decreased spontaneous nystagmus and decreased slow phase velocity of OKR nystagmus.

Table II. Effect of hyperventilation on speed of slow component and frequency of optokinetic nystagmus in pathological subjects without spontaneous nystagmus

Patient No.	SSC	Frequency	Pathology
9	---	*	central
10	*	++	periph.
11	*	*	central/periph.
12	--	−	periph.
13	*	*	periph.
14	*	++	periph.

SSC = Speed of slow component; * = unchanged; −/+ = <10%; −−/++ = 10–20%; −−−/+++ = >20%.

significantly and constantly enhanced by hyperventilation at least in normal subjects. Furthermore, preliminary observations on pathological subjects demonstrate that hyperventilation may exert some influence on the quantitative characteristics of nystagmus, either spontaneous or optokinetically induced, although this influence, at present, cannot be defined in satisfactorily interpretable terms. Since it appears very likely that hyperventilation produces similar effects on nystagmic responses induced by acceleratory stimuli, it may be concluded, first of all, that we are in the presence of a phenomenon which deserves to be extensively studied, both in relation to its physiological significance and to its potentialities as a useful tool for clinical investigation.

It must be pointed out that hyperventilation does not produce, in itself, any nystagmus in normal subjects. It only influences, by enhancing them, the quantitative characteristics of normal responses. It must act, therefore, on some of the mechanisms which are responsible for the modulation of the automatic brain stem reflex, and which usually tend to exert some kind of inhibition on it, thus decreasing the reflex gain. The cerebellar vestibular cortex may be a likely candidate. On the other hand, on the presently available premises, if it is true that hyperventilation acts through the mechanism of hypercapnia – decrease in blood pH, vasoconstriction – on the cortical structures, which may be more sensitive to the reduction in the pressure of O_2, some action on the efferent control system may also be postulated. On many grounds, including insufficiency of available data, the problem cannot be discussed exhaustively here.

From a clinical point of view, hyperventilation seems likely to provide some useful contribution to a better evaluation of the quantitative characteristics of the nystagmic response in any clinically possible condition, very likely also of responses obtained from patients suffering from peripheral labyrinthine disturbances. Individual and interindividual variability of quantitative characteristics may be significantly reduced by hyperventilation, thus making responses more homogeneous, reproducible and meaningful for diagnostic purposes. The absence of the effect itself may prove to be clinically significant as seems to be suggested by a preliminary analysis of our pathologic cases. In the presence of lesions of the CNS, the situation is, as expected, far more complicated. Our results indicate, at present, that hyperventilation produces in most cases some effect in the characteristics of the nystagmus. Interpreting the mechanism of these changes is even more difficult, not sufficiently substantiated at present, but deserving of further investigation.

References

1 Carpenter, D. O.; Hubbard, J. H.; Humphrey, D.R.; Thomson, H.K.; Marshall, W.H.: Carbon dioxide effects on nerve cell fraction; in Nahas, Schaeffer, Carbon dioxide and metabolic regulations (Springer, New York 1974).
2 Drachman, D.A.; Hart, C.W.: An approach to the dizzy patient. Neurology 22: 323–334 (1972).
3 Gotoh, F.; Meyer, J.S.; Takagi, Y.: Cerebral effects of hyperventilation in man. Archs Neurol. 12: 410–423 (1965).
4 Krnjevic, K.; Randic, M.; Siesjo, B.K.: Cortical CO_2-tension and neuronal excitability. J. Physiol. 176: 102–122 (1965).
5 Monday, L.A.; Tetreault, L.: Hyperventilation and vertigo. Laryngoscope 90: 1003–1010 (1980).
6 Rosignoli, M.; Almadori, G.; Maurizi, M.: Effetti della iperventilazione volontaria sul nistagmo perrotatorio. Acta otorhinol. ital. 4: 667–677 (1984).
7 Theunissen, E.J.J.M.; Huygen, P.L.M.; Folgering, H.T.: Vestibular hyperreactivity and hyperventilation. Clin. Otolaryngol. 11: 161–169 (1986).

G.C. Modugno, MD, Clinica Otorinolaringologica dell'Università di Bologna,
Via Massarenti 9, I-40138 Bologna (Italy)

Adv. Oto-Rhino-Laryng., vol. 42, pp. 116–122 (Karger, Basel 1988)

C3 and C1q Complement Deposits in the Membranous Labyrinth of Patients with Ménière's Disease

Rudolf Häusler[a], *Wolfgang Arnold*[b], *Jürg Schifferli*[c]

[a]Clinic of Otolaryngology, Head and Neck Surgery, Cantonal University Hospital, Geneva; [b]Clinic of Otolaryngology, Head and Neck Surgery, Cantonal Hospital, Lucerne; [c]Department of Medicine, Cantonal University Hospital, Geneva, Switzerland

The hypothesis that certain types of inner ear dysfunctions are generated through immunopathological mechanisms has been advocated for at least 30 years [1, 3, 11, 12, 14]. Several recent studies suggest that immunological reactions may also play an important role in Ménière's disease. Clinical case reports indicate that favourable effects on hearing and on vertigo have been obtained with steroid therapy and immunosuppression in some patients with Ménière's disease [5, 8, 9, 23, 24]. Other investigations report the presence of circulating immune complexes and antibodies against inner ear structures in patients with Ménière's disease [2, 5, 23]. Finally, experimental studies demonstrate that it is possible to produce autoimmune mediated endolymphatic hydrops in animals [8, 22, 23].

The interesting results of these studies have led us to perform immunohistochemical examinations on membranous labyrinth structures of 2 patients who had suffered from an advanced Ménière's disease. The inner ear fragments have been obtained in these patients by labyrinthectomy which had become unavoidable for the 2 unilaterally deaf patients in order to relieve them from disabling vestibular symptoms.

Patients

Patient A, born in 1943, is a middle-aged healthy man who had suffered during his childhood from bilateral chronic otitis media. Central tympanic perforations persisted in adult age; however, there were, for many years, no more signs of ear infection. At the age of 33, he noted for the first time an intermittent tinnitus in his right ear and he began to develop a fluctuating right hearing loss. At irregular intervals he also suffered from vertigo attacks. Between age 40 and 43 he had at least two dizzy spells a week and, in addition, he had frequent falling attacks without loss of consciousness. Between 1982 and 1986 the hearing in his right ear had deteriorated progressively to profound deafness. Caloric examination was normal in both ears.

We concluded that the patient had a severe form of Ménière's disease in his right ear. In order to relieve him from his disabling vestibular symptoms, a transmeatal, transtapedial labyrinthectomy was performed in May 1986. Before removing the stapes, inner ear liquid was sampled with a Silverstein micropipette through a small puncture of the footplate [18]. On quantitative analysis by flame emission photometry a potassium level twice that of sodium was measured indicating the presence of an advanced endolymphatic hydrops up to the stapes footplate [16]. The membranous inner ear structures were extracted with a hook and fixed in Bouin's solution for histological examination. After the operation the patient exhibited for a few days the signs of an acute right vestibular deficit. Afterwards, he had no new dizziness attacks and he never had another falling attack.

Patient B, born in 1938, is a healthy middle-aged woman with absence of hearing in her left ear known since her early childhood. Since the age of 40, she had several vertigo attacks with nausea and vomiting. During the 9 months prior to her admission she complained of constant disabling disequilibrium. The pure tone audiogram indicated normal hearing thresholds in her right ear and confirmed the absence of hearing in her left ear. Caloric examination was normal in both ears. We concluded that she had in her non-hearing ear a particular form of Ménière's disease reported as 'delayed endolymphatic hydrops' [17].

A transmeatal labyrinthectomy was performed in September 1986. The examined inner ear liquid, aspirated directly under the stapes footplate, again showed a concentration of potassium which was severalfold higher than that of sodium as a sign for the presence of an endolymphatic hydrops [16, 18]. This patient, too, was definitively relieved from her vestibular symptoms after the operation.

The following blood tests were all normal or negative in both patients: ESR, haemoglobin, white blood cells, platelets, immunoelectrophoresis, immunoglobulins G, A and M, complement (C3, C4, CH50, C3d), CRP, cryoglobulins, Latex, antistreptolysine, Coombs's test, VDRL and TPHA, C1q binding test for immune complexes, and various autoantibodies (antinuclear, antidouble-stranded DNA, antimitochondrial, antigastric parietal cell, antismooth muscle, antimicrosomal and antithyroglobulin), HBS Ag and Ab.

Materials and Methods

The extracted membranous inner ear structures of the 2 labyrinthectomized patients which had been fixed in Bouin's solution were embedded in paraffin, and cut into 4-μm sections.

After deparaffinization, immunohistochemistry was performed according to Bourne [4] using peroxidase-conjugated antibodies against human IgG, IgA, IgM and complement C3 (Dako Corporation products). Immunofluorescence was performed using fluoresceinated antibodies against human complement C1q.

For control, identical methods were applied to sections from six healthy temporal bones which had been removed from persons without hearing problems shortly after death. (The immunohistochemical reactions were kindly performed with the help of the Pathology Department of the Cantonal Hospital in Lucerne.)

Results

The immunohistochemically investigated parts of the membranous labyrinth showed in both patients well recognizable deposits of complement C3 and C1q along the basement membrane (fig. 1a, c). For C3 there were in some areas patchy deposits within the subepithelial connective tissue. Adjacent control sections of each patient treated with peroxidase only (that is without antibodies against human C3) were all negative.

In the control specimens of normal labyrinthine structures treated with the same methods no complement deposits were seen (fig. 1b). Immunoglobulin deposits IgG, IgA and IgM were not detected in the 2 patients examined, nor in the controls (table I).

Discussion

This study provides clear evidence for complement deposition on membranous labyrinthine structures in 2 patients exhibiting endolymphatic hydrops and suffering from Ménière's symptomatology. In the absence of any systemic disease, such as diabetes or a recent general or local infection, these findings could well indicate that an immunopathological process had taken place in the inner ears of these patients.

Two mechanisms leading to complement depositions along basement membranes could be involved. First, an antibody could react with an antigen located in or near the basement membrane. This binding would be responsible for local complement activation and deposition (fig. 2a). This type of antibody-mediated reaction is known to occur in antiglomerular basement membrane antibody disease (Goodpasture's syndrome), pemphigoid and herpes gestationis [10, 15, 21].

Second, antibodies may react with soluble antigens of an exogenous or endogenous nature. These immune complexes may be deposited along basement membranes where complement activation would take place (fig. 2b). There is evidence that this type of immune complex deposition occurs in

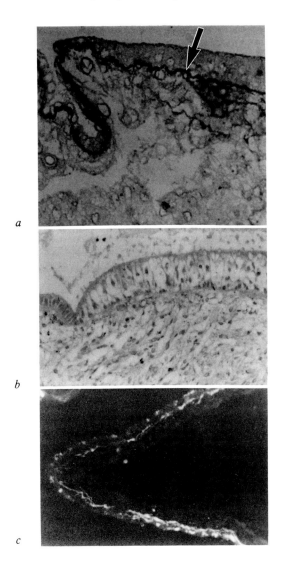

Fig. 1. Immunohistochemistry and immunofluorescence on membranous inner ear fragments. *a* The arrow indicates C3 deposits along an inner ear basement membrane (presumably utricular) from patient A suffering from a typical Ménière's disease. The sensory epithelium (region of the arrow) has a partially degenerated aspect. Similar results have been obtained in patient B suffering from a 'delayed endolymphatic hydrops'. *b* Absence of C3 deposits in a utricular fragment of a control. *c* C1q deposits along inner ear basement membrane from patient A (immunofluorescence). Similar results have been obtained in patient B.

Table I. Immunohistochemical results on membranous inner ear structures

	With endolymphatic hydrops		Controls (n L 6)
	patient A	patient B	
IgA	–	–	–
IgG	–	–	–
IgM	–	–	–
C1q	+ [1]	+ [1]	–
C3	+ [1]	+ [1]	–

[1] Along inner ear basement membranes (presumably utricular).

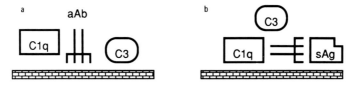

Basement membrane

Fig. 2. Immunopathological mechanisms leading to complement deposition along basement membranes. *a* Autoantibody-mediated. Autoantibodies (aAb) acting against basement membrane antigens may lead to local complement activation (C1q, C3) (example: Goodpasture's syndrome). *b* Immune complex deposition-mediated. Antibodies acting against soluble antigens (sAg) may be deposited along basement membranes and activate complement (example: systemic lupus erythematosus). Either of the two mechanisms might apply to the inner ear basement membrane complement deposits found in the 2 patients with Ménière's disease reported here.

systemic lupus erythematosus along basement membranes of skin and glomeruli [7, 13].

Either of the two mechanisms may apply to the inner ear basement membrane complement deposits observed in our 2 patients with Ménière's disease. The fact that no IgA, IgG or IgM were detected in our specimens should not detract from an antibody-dependent reaction, since immunoglobulins may be masked by heavy complement deposits [10].

As a working hypothesis for an immunopathological origin of Ménière's disease we suggest that, following a non-specific local insult (e.g. of infectious or traumatic nature) to the inner ear, immunocompetent cells become sensitized to specific labyrinthine structures. A local antigen antibody reaction occurring in the inner ear would activate complement proteins and lead to the observed linear deposits along the basement membranes. It is known that such complement deposits can damage membrane permeability [6]. Disturbed membrane permeability — either because of leakage or because of a permeability blockage — could lead to the buildup of an endolymphatic hydrops and in parallel produce the clinical symptoms of Ménière's disease.

References

1   Arnold, W.; Weidauer, H.; Seelig, H.P.: Experimenteller Beweis einer gemeinsamen Antigenizität zwischen Innenohr und Niere. Archs Otolar. *212:* 99–106 (1976).
2   Arnold, W.; Pfaltz, R.; Altermatt, H.J.: Evidence of serum antibodies against inner ear tissues in the blood of patients with certain sensorineural hearing disorders. Acta oto-lar. *99:* 437–444 (1985).
3   Beickert. V.P.: Zur Frage der Empfindungsschwerhörigkeit unter Autoallergie. Z. Lar. Rhinol. Otol. *40:* 837–842 (1961).
4   Bourne, J.A.: Handbook of immunoperoxidase staining methods (Dako Corp., Santa Barbara 1983).
5   Brookes, G.B.: Circulating immune complexes in Ménière's disease. Archs Otolar. *112:* 536–540 (1986).
6   Couser, W.G.; Baker, P.J.; Adler, S.: Complement and the direct mediation of immune glomerular injury: a new perspective. Kidney int. *28:* 879–890 (1985).
7   Gilliam, J.N.: Systemic lupus erythematosus and the skin; in Lahita, Systemic lupus erythematosus, vol. 23, pp. 615–642 (Wiley & Sons, New York 1987).
8   Harris, J.P.: Experimental autoimmune sensorineural hearing loss. Laryngoscope *97:* 63–76 (1987).
9   Hughes, G.B.; Kinney, S.E.; Barna, B.P.: Autoimmune reactivity in Ménière's disease: a preliminary report. Laryngoscope *93:* 410–417 (1983).
10 Katz, S.I.; Hertz, K.C.; Yaoita, H.: Herpes gestationis: immunopathology and characterization of the HG factor. J. clin. Invest. *57:* 1434–1441 (1976).
11 Kikuchi, M.: On the 'sympathetic otitis'. Zibi Rinsyo Kyoto *52:* 600–605 (1959).
12 Lehnardt, E.: Plötzliche Hörstörungen auf beiden Seiten gleichzeitig oder nacheinander aufgetreten. Z. Lar. Rhinol. Otol. *37:* 1 (1958).
13 Mannik, M.: Immune complexes; in Lahita, Systemic lupus erythematosus, vol. 12, pp. 333–351 (Wiley & Sons, New York 1987).
14 McCabe, B.F.: Autoimmune sensorineural hearing loss. Ann. Otol. Rhinol. Lar. *88:* 585–589 (1979).
15 Muhlemann, M.F.; Cream, J.J.: Bullous diseases. Clin. Immunol. Allergy *5:* 601–612 (1985).
16 Schuknecht, H.F.: Pathology of the ear, pp. 151–153, 463–464 (Harvard University Press, Cambridge 1974).
17 Schuknecht, H.F.: Delayed endolymphatic hydrops. Ann. Otol. Rhinol. Lar. *87:* 743–748 (1978).
18 Silverstein. H.; Griffin, W.: Diagnostic labyrinthotomy in otologic disorders. Archs Otolar. *91:* 414–423 (1970).

19 Terayama, Y.; Sasaki, Y.: Studies on experimental allergic (isoimmune) labyrinthitis in guinea pigs. Acta oto-lar. *58:* 49–64 (1964).
20 Williams, L.L.; Lowery, H.W.; Shannon, B.T.: Evidence of persistent viral infection in Ménière's disease. Archs Otolar. *113:* 397–400 (1987).
21 Williams, D.G.; Peters, D.K.: The immunology of nephritis; in Lachmann, Peters, Clinical aspects of immunology, vol. 29, pp. 853–877 (Blackwell, Oxford 1982).
22 Woolf, N.K.; Haris, J.: Cochlear pathophysiology associated with inner ear immune responses. Acta oto-lar. *102:* 353–364 (1986).
23 Yoo, T.J.: Etiopathogenesis of Ménière's disease: a hypothesis. Ann. Otol. Rhinol. Lar. *93:* suppl. 113, pp. 6–12 (1984).
24 Yoo, T.J.: Autoimmune disorders of the cochlea; in Altschuler, Hoffman, Bobbin, Neurobiology of hearing, pp. 425–440 (Raven Press, New York 1986).

R. Häusler, MD, Clinic of Otolaryngology, Head and Neck Surgery,
Cantonal University Hospital, CH-1211 Geneva 4 (Switzerland)

Adv. Oto-Rhino-Laryng., vol. 42, pp. 123–128 (Karger, Basel 1988)

Immunohistochemical Localization of Na⁺-K⁺-ATPase in the Endolymphatic Sac

Hideo Yamane, Yoshiaki Nakai

Department of Otolaryngology, Osaka City University Medical School, Abeno, Osaka, Japan

Introduction

Many authors have described that the dynamic balance of inner ear fluid is maintained primarily by the stria vascularis and endolymphatic sac (ES) [2–4], and it is said that endolymphatic hydrops is due to disturbance of this balance, which is associated with various factors, such as Ménière's disease, fluctuant hearing loss, and vertigo [6]. Recently, some interesting studies were presented, which suggested that passive absorption of K^+ and endolymph occurs in the endolymphatic duct (ED) [5, 7], not only in the ES as postulated earlier. In the meantime, an enzyme histochemical investigation demonstrated some enzymes in the ES which supposedly play a role in the transport of ions and fluid [8]. However, enzyme histochemical methods in general have some problems in specificity. In this work we could locate Na^+-K^+-ATPase in the ES by immunohistochemical techniques.

Materials and Methods

Eight pigmented guinea pigs weighing 250–350 g were used. Under sodium pentobarbital anesthesia they were decapitated and the ES including the ED were collected and immersed in 4% paraformaldehyde in 0.1 M phosphate-buffered saline (PBS). Ultrathin sections (10 µm in thickness) were prepared in a cryostat at −20 °C and studied by the immunofluorescence method and the avidin-biotin-peroxidase complex (ABC) method. These sections were incubated with goat anti-Na^+-K^+-ATPase antibody (Clark Laboratories Inc.) diluted 1:50 or 1:100 in PBS. For fluorescence immunohistochemistry these sections were further treated with fluorescein isocyanate (FITC)-conjugated rabbit anti-

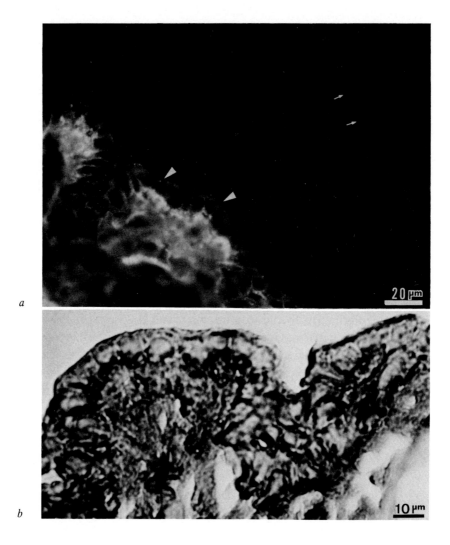

Fig. 1. a Distribution of Na⁺-K⁺-ATPase in the intermediate part of the ES. This enzyme is seen chiefly along the basolateral membrane of the epithelium. The fluorescence intensity is stronger at the epithelium facing the sigmoid sinus (arrowheads) than at the epithelium on the opposite side or on the side of the cerebellum (small arrows). Immunofluorescence. *b* Distribution of Na⁺-K⁺-ATPase in the kidney (positive control). ABC method.

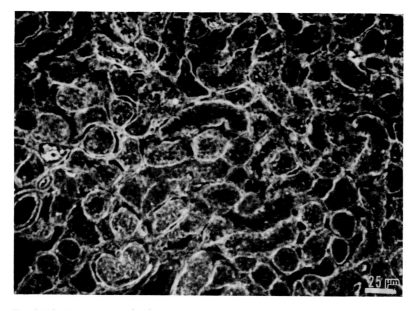

Fig. 2. Distribution of Na⁺-K⁺-ATPase in the kidney (positive control). The enzyme is present mainly along the basolateral membrane of distal tubules. Immunofluorescence.

goat antibody (Miles) diluted 1:50 or 1:100 in PBS. In a negative control experiment the first serum was replaced by normal goat serum or was omitted. In a positive control experiment the kidney of the same animal was used instead of the ES.

Results

Na⁺-K⁺-ATPase was detected along the basolateral membrane of the epithelium of the ES, mainly in the proximal to intermediate portion, whichever method might be concerned (fig. 1a, b). The epithelium facing the sigmoid sinus was relatively rich in this enzyme (fig. 1a). In the kidney, as a positive control, this enzyme was located at the basolateral membrane of renal tubules (fig. 2). No fluorescence was detected in the negative control (fig. 3).

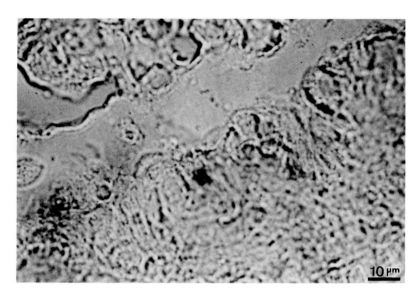

Fig. 3. Negative control of the ES. Na$^+$-K$^+$-ATPase is absent. ABC method.

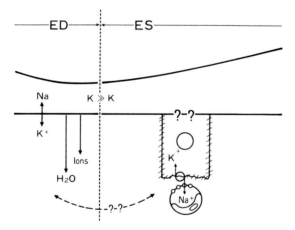

Fig. 4. Schema showing K$^+$transport in the ES (drawn after that presented by Rask-Andersen et al. [5] with a modification). The source of K$^+$ exists outside of the basolateral membrane of the ES epithelium (oblique lines).

Discussion

Regulation of ion composition in the endolymph has been thought to occur primarily at the stria vascularis and the ED or ES. Also, the low level of K$^+$ in the ES makes a sharp contrast with the high level in the cochlear duct. This difference may be explained by the persuasive hypothesis based on the ultramorphological observation that the K$^+$ of the ES is absorbed by the ED [5]. However, the present observation that Na$^+$-K$^+$-ATPase relating to ion and fluid transport existed in the ES, especially along the basolateral membrane of the epithelium facing the sigmoid sinus, might suggest that Na$^+$, K$^+$ and fluid transport is regulated not only by the ED but also by the ES, and support the overview about inner ear fluid transport which was presented by Vosteen and Morgenstern [8].

Generally speaking, the tissues which have a luminal structure transport ions and fluid by the aid of Na$^+$-K$^+$-ATPase, which commonly exists along the basolateral membrane of epithelial cells. Ernst et al [1] found this enzyme in the choroid plexus which is morphologically similar to the ES. More specifically, it was localized on the luminal side of the epithelium. They also discussed this peculiar localization in comparison with that in other tissues. They further discussed the availability of an immunohistochemical method as compared with an enzyme histochemical method, and postulated that the former might be more reliable. The present study, in which we used negative and positive controls, produced data in support of this postulate.

The exact role of the ES or ED in the regulation of inner ear fluid is yet to be elucidated. In consideration of the nature of Na$^+$-K$^+$-ATPase, the source of K$^+$ must be outside of the basolateral membrane of the ES (fig.4), though no definite evidence has been obtained hitherto. More intensive studies have to be carried out to clarify the precise localization of this and any other enzyme involved in inner ear fluid transport, for the eventual purpose of better managing patients with endolymphatic hydrops, a disease resulting from the dynamic imbalance of inner ear fluid.

References

1   Ernst, S.A.; Palacios, I.I., Jr.; Siegel, G.J.: Immunocytochemical localization of Na$^+$, K$^+$-ATPase catalytic polypeptide in mouse choroid plexus. J. Histochem. Cytochem. *34:* 189–195 (1986).
2   Guild, S.R.: The circulation of the endolymph. Am. J. Anat. *39:* 57–81 (1927).

3   Kimura, R.S.; Schuknecht, H.F.: Membranous hydrops in the inner ear of the guinea pigs after obliteration of the endolymphatic sac. Practica oto-rhino-lar. *27:* 343–354 (1965).
4   Konishi, T.: Effect of ouabain on cochlear potentials and endolymph composition in guinea pigs. Acta oto-lar. *69:* 192–199 (1970).
5   Rask-Andersen, H.; Bredberg, G.; Stahle, J.: Structure and function of the endolymphatic duct; in Vosteen, Schuknecht, Pfaltz, Versäll, Kimura, Morgenstern, Juhn, Ménière's disease. Pathogenesis, diagnosis and treatment, pp. 127–140 (Thieme, Stuttgart 1980).
6   Schuknecht, H.F.: Pathology of the ear (Harvard University Press, Cambridge 1974).
7   Stahle, J.; Wilbrand, H.: The vestibular aqueduct in patients with Ménière's disease. Acta oto-lar. *78:* 36–48 (1974).
8   Vosteen, K.H.; Morgenstern, C.: Biochemical aspect of inner ear pathology; in Pfaltz, Controversial aspects of Ménière's disease, pp. 16–28 (Thieme, Stuttgart 1986).

Hideo Yamane, MD, Department of Otolaryngology, Osaka City
University Medical School, Abeno Osaka 545 (Japan)

Adv. Oto-Rhino-Laryng., vol. 42, pp. 129–134 (Karger, Basel 1988)

Immunohistochemical Analysis of the Lateral Wall of the Endolymphatic Sac in Ménière's Patients
(with one color plate)

Takashi Futaki, Yumiko Nagao, Shigeru Kikuchi

Department of Otolaryngology, University of Tokyo, Tokyo, Japan

Introduction

The function of the endolymphatic sac is understood to be mainly resorption of endolymph, according to the 'longitudinal theory' [1]. We were able to obtain and analyze a very small amount of human intra-sac endolymph and the small specimen of the lateral wall during the lateral wall turning procedure [2].

From the efflux of endolymph resorption in the endolymphatic duct, we could determine, as previously reported [3], that the specific value of IgG concentration is higher in patients with Ménière's disease than in controls. It is well known that a high gradient of IgG can be recognized at the site of the lesion in many autoimmunological diseases. This finding might mean that autoimmunological mechanisms have operated somewhere in the endolymphatic lumen and caused the hydrops.

As a follow-up to this 'humoral' study of intra-sac endolymph, immunohistochemical analysis of the lateral wall itself should be undertaken to obtain further information which would make progress toward revealing the genetic cause of endolymphatic hydrops.

Materials and Methods

Two sets of specimens were prepared. One set, analyzed by luminescent microscopy, consisted of the lateral walls of the endolymphatic sac of 9 patients with Ménière's disease and one acoustic tumor as a negative control.

The other set, analyzed by the avidin-biotin-peroxidase-complex method (ABC method) described below, consisted of lateral walls from 4 Ménière's patients and one from a case of delayed endolymphatic hydrops (DEH). During ELS surgery, the smallest possible area of the corner of the L-shaped incised lateral wall was carefully held by a small clamp in order to avoid tissue damage, and cut off using a sharp cornea mess. Into the space of the removed lateral wall, triple-folded, triangle-shaped gelatine films were inserted toward the ductus endolymphaticus. Immediately after the specimen was cut off, it was frozen with thin OCT compound paste in hexane of $-70\,°C$ surrounded by dry ice blocks in acetone for the luminescence method. Five specimens were fixed in a buffered 2% formalin solution for paraffin sectioning. As positive controls, small pieces of tonsil were frozen and fixed in the same way as the sac specimens.

Methods

(1) Luminescent microscopy using fluorescein isocyanate (FITC)-labeled antihuman IgA, IgG, IgM, IgE, C_{1q}, C_3, C_4 and fibrinogen (goat) (Hoechst Co. Ltd) applied to the frozen sections without any fixation. In order to preserve the antigenic titer in the specimen, no fixation was applied to the specimens for luminescence investigation. The cutting direction of the cryostat was set at a right angle to the epithelial layer of the inner surface. These frozen sections on the glass were dried in an ordinary refrigerator at $-4\,°C$ overnight. After blocking for nonspecific binding by the diluted standard human serum and washing by phosphate-buffered saline (PBS), sections were incubated for 1 h at 38 °C in a dark wet chamber, and then washed and covered with a drop of glycerin. The sections were inspected and photodocumented in an ultraviolet microscope.

(2) Light microscopy using biotinized antihuman IgG and IgM stained by the ABC method. Subsequent to the routine procedures for paraffin sections, the samples were incubated in methanol with 0.3% H_2O_2 and blocked to the nonspecific binding sites by diluted standard serum. Two incubation steps were performed, one by biotinized antihuman IgG and IgM (goat, $X10^2$) for 30 min at 37 °C, the other by the ABC method for 30 min at 37 °C. The sections were inspected after coloring by DAB and H_2O_2 solution.

Results

Fluorescein-Labeled Antiserum Method

The section (fig. 1) was a sample stained with FITC-conjugated antihuman IgG and fibrinogen (fig. 2); the bright apple-green fluorescence shown as 'lumpy bumpy' or 'nebulosity' indicates antibody deposits in the epithelial layer or subepithelial space.

Table I gives the results of this series. (+) indicates positive immunofluorescence and (–), negative. Except for the positive rate of fibrinogen, the highest in the Ménière's patients was that of IgG (83%), followed by IgA (63%) and IgM (38%) in immunoglobulin. In the positive control tonsil, the result was also positive for these four items. The results for negative control AT in immunoglobulin, however, were negative.

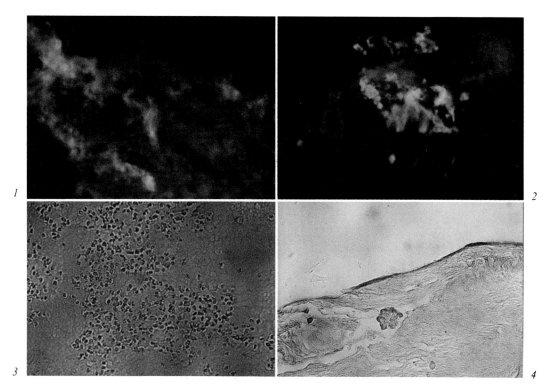

Fig. 1. An immunofluorescence by FITC-conjugated antihuman IgG. The bright apple-green fluorescence shown as 'lumpy bumpy' indicates antihuman IgG deposits in the lateral wall of the sac.

Fig. 2. The one by antihuman fibrinogen.

Fig. 3. The positive control of the tonsil stained by biotinized IgG. Brown deposit of IgG could be seen in the lymphocytes and the plasma cells.

Fig. 4. The inner surface of the lateral wall of the sac reacted by the ABC method. The brown precipitation of biotinized IgG can be investigated in the epithelial cell layer and the subepithelial crypt (arrow).

Table I. The results of immunofluorescence

Specimen No.	FITC-labeled antihuman							
	IgA	IgG	IgM	C_1q	C_3	C_4	Fibrinogen	IgE
1	+	+	+	−	+	+	+	
3	+		+	−			−	+
5			+		−	−	+	
6	−		−		−		+	
7	+	+	−	−	−	−	+	
8	−	+	−		+		+	
9	+	+	−	−	−	−	+	−
10	+	+	−	−	+	−	+	−
11	−	−	−	−	−	−	+	−
Positive rate:	5/8 (63%)	5/6 (83%)	3/8 (38%)	0/7	3/8 (38%)	0/7	9/9 (100%)	0/3
Control of AT	−	−	−	−	−	−	+	−
Tonsil	+	+	+	−	−	−	+	−

+ = Positive fluorescence.

Investigation of IgG and IgM by ABC method

In the positive control tonsil, brown deposits of IgG could be seen in the lymphocytes and the plasma cells (fig. 3). Inspection of the inner surface of the lateral wall of the sac revealed the brown precipitation of biotinized IgG in the epithelial cell layer and the subepithelial crypt (fig. 4).

The surgical findings and the immunohistochemical results for the 5 patients were given in table II; (+) indicates the distinct existence of a complex deposit in the right two columns.

Three out of 5 patients showed positive for IgG, but only one was positive for IgM. There was no relationship between sedimentation and the size or grade of fibrosis of the sac; however, in the 2 patients who could be inspected for seepage of endolymph, deposits could not be found in the epithelium.

Discussion

McCabe [4] proposed the existence of autoimmune sensorineural hearing loss in 18 patients, in one of whom a vasculitis was evident. Yoo et al. [5]

Table II. The results of ABC method

	Size of the sac	Fibrosis (+++ −)	Seepage of endolymph	Deposit of	
				IgG	IgM
1	middle	++	no	+	−
2	small	+++	no	+	−
3	large	++	yes	−	−
4	large	+	yes	−	−
5	large	+	no	+	+

described an animal model of immunologically mediated hearing loss, i.e. hypersensitivity to native type II collagen, and suggested [6] that Ménière's might include autoimmunity to collagen in its genetic makeup. Shea [7] also reported that steroid-reacting hearing loss had an autoimmunological genesis. Rask-Andersen and Stahle [8] reported that the endolymphatic duct is concerned with fluid resorption while the sac is engaged in phagocytosis and acts as an immunodefensive organ for the internal ear.

Prior to this paper, Guild [1] described floating cells in the lumen; Yamakawa [9] reported 'Sekretmassen' in the sac; Andersen [10] proposed that it is the task of the intrasaccular cells to clear away a large amount of protein-like substance; and Engström and Hjorth [11] reported that the major part of the dye is localized in the intrasaccular cells and that the rugose portion and perisaccular tissue contain histiocytes; Arnvig [12] showed that the vessels of the perisaccular connective tissue of the intermediate part do not contain blood but a fluid rich in proteins and white blood corpuscles at work in the decomposition of the high molecular proteins; Lundquist et al. [13] reported that the most active part of the sac and duct was the intermediate portion, where pinocytosis appeared to be a main function; and Ishii et al. [14] hypothesized that the sac is a metabolically active structure where proteins are phagocytized and/or transported via the lining epithelial cells into the perisaccular connective tissue. All these papers were reports of animal experiments. In humans, a few studies have been reported, for example Hallpike and Cairns [15] and Zechner and Altmann [16] who demonstrated the diminishing of perisaccular connective tissue in Ménière's patients.

The present authors determined the specific value of IgG concentration to be higher in Ménière's than in a control using the intra-sac endolymph through an immunological assay of microanalysis of the proteins [3]. This finding might mean that some immunological disorders occurred in the endolymphatic lumen, albeit in an unspecified location.

This sufficient production of IgG might be related to the possibility of (1) an active infiltration of plasma cells, (2) an increase in the permeability of the cell membrane adjacent to the endolymphatic space, or (3) an increase in phagocytic activity and lymphocyte agglutination in some part of the endo-lymphatic system. To follow up this 'humoral' finding, we intended to obtain immunohistochemical results in the human material of the Ménière's patients and a control as the first step.

As in the results of the immunofluorescent procedure, the deposit or precipitation showed the highest positive rate in IgG (83%), second highest in IgA (63%), in the third in IgM (38%) in the epithelial cells or subepithelial crypt. This high gradient deposition of IgG in the epithelial region of the sac might correspond to the high concentration of IgG in the intra-sac endolymph.

Yamane et al. [17] reported similar precipitation of IgG in the epithe-lium and the subepithelial part of the sac in the guinea pig. In humans, Arnold et al. [18] found no positive reaction to IgG or IgA, and a positive reaction only to IgM on the epithelial membrane and on the epithelial surface of the intermediate part of the sac of fresh human specimens. There is no clear statement that these specimens were from Ménière's patients. Our results in a control with IgG, IgA and IgM have not yielded positive reactions. In Ménière's patients, IgG deposition in the sac might be a characteristic feature in the immunohistochemical results.

The disadvantage of luminescent-microscopic investigation, as is well known, is the difficulty of discrete identification of the reaction site in the tissue. In order to obtain more concrete histological information about immunological deposition, the ABC method was used on the five specimens of the sac. The brown particles of deposits could be found in the cytoplasm of the epithelium cells and agglutination in the subepithelial space. IgG was positive in 3 out of 5, IgM in only 20%. In the 2 patients with negative IgG, the seepage of the endolymph immediately after the opening incision of the sac was inspected.

In these cases, there might not be sufficient retardation of the intra-sac flow as to justify carrying out pinocytic precipitation of immunoglobulin toward the epithelium. The results obtained by two kinds of immunohisto-chemical procedures might be interpreted as follows: some immunological disorder may occur which raises the IgG concentration in the upper space of the endolymphatic lumen from the duct to the cochlea and which results in its deposition on the wall of the sac, or some change in phagocytotic activity of the sac itself might take place which would increase the remaining IgG. These results may have a close relationship to the immunological disorder which causes endolymphatic hydrops of the labyrinth.

References

1 Guild, S.R.: The circulation of the endolymph. Am. J. Anat. *39:* 57–81 (1927).
2 Kitahara, M.; Futaki, T.; et al.: Epidural operation for Ménière's disease. Int. J. Equilib. Res. *4:* 48–51 (1974).
3 Futaki, T.; et al.: Immunological analysis of IgG and other protein fractions in endolymph obtained from endolymphatic sac of Ménière's patients and a control. Acta oto-lar., suppl. 419, pp. 71–78 (1985).
4 McCabe, B.F.: Autoimmune sensorineural hearing loss. Ann. Otol. Rhinol. Lar. *88:* 585–589 (1979).
5 Yoo, T.J.; et al.: Type II collagen-induced autoimmune sensorineural hearing loss and vestibular dysfunction in rats. Ann. Otol. Rhinol. Lar. *92:* 267–271 (1983).
6 Yoo, T.J.; et al.: Type II collagen autoimmunity in otosclerosis and Ménière's disease. Science *217:* 1153–1155 (1982).
7 Shea, J.J.: Autoimmune sensorineural hearing loss as an aggravating factor in Ménière's disease. Adv. Oto-Rhino-Laryng., vol. 30, pp. 254–257 (Karger, Basel 1983).
8 Rask-Andersen, H.; Stahle, J.: Immunodefence of the inner ear? Lymphocyte-macrophage interaction in the endolymphatic sac. Acta oto-lar. *89:* 283–290 (1980).
9 Yamakawa, K.: Die Wirkung der arsenigen Säure auf das Ohr. Arch. Orh.-Nas.-KehlkHeilk. *123:* 238–296 (1929).
10 Andersen, H.C.: Passage of trypan blue into the endolymphatic system of the labyrinth. Acta oto-lar. *36:* 273–283 (1948).
11 Engström, H.; Hjorth, S.: On the distribution and localization of injected dyes in the labyrinth of the guinea pig. Acta oto-lar., suppl. 95, pp. 149–158 (1950).
12 Arnvig, J.: Lymph vessels in the wall of the endolymphatic sac. Archs Otolar. *53:* 290–295 (1951).
13 Lundquist, P.G.; et al.: Ultrastructural organization of the epithelial lining in the endolymphatic duct and sac in the guinea pig. Acta oto-lar. *57:* 65–80 (1964).
14 Ishii, T.; et al.: Metabolic activities of the endolymphatic sac. Acta oto-lar. *62:* 61–72 (1969).
15 Hallpike, C.S.; Cairns, H.: Observation on the pathology of Ménière's syndrome. J. Laryngol. *53:* 625–655 (1938).
16 Zechner, G.; Altmann, F.: Histologic studies on the human endolymphatic duct and sac. Practica oto-rhino-lar. *31:* 65–83 (1969).
17 Yamane, H.; et al.: Distribution of immunoglobulin in the endolymphatic sac of the guinea pig. Ear Res. Jap. *17:* 215–219 (1986).
18 Arnold, W.; et al.: Morphology and function of the endolymphatic sac; in Vosteen, Ménière's disease, pp. 110–114 (Thieme, Stuttgart 1981).

Takashi Futaki, MD, Department of Otolaryngology, University of Tokyo,
7-3-1 Hongo, Bunkyo-ku, Tokyo 113 (Japan)

Adv. Oto-Rhino-Laryng., vol. 42, pp. 135–138 (Karger, Basel 1988)

Considerations on Vestibular Physiopathology with Special Reference to Comparison of Irritative State and Paralytic State

J. Hozawa, K. Ishikawa, F. Fukuoka, S. Ohta

Department of Otolargyngology, Hirosaki University School of Medicine, Hirosaki, Japan

Introduction

Irritative nystagmus (I-ny) directs to the side of the impared labyrinth, and paralytic nystagmus (P-ny) directs to the contralateral side. This fact has been well known by many experiments and clinical researches. However, the detailed analysis of differences between the two characteristic types of nystagmus has not been reported. The purpose of this paper is to clarify the characteristic differences and to consider the vestibular physiopathological mechanism of the two types of nystagmus.

Materials and Methods

Experimental Study
Potassium ion was introduced through the round window into the right perilymphatic space of 40 guinea pigs by means of iontophoresis, and the influence of the high perilymphatic potassium concentration was investigated physiologically and histochemically, namely the changing process of the provoked nystagmus was observed by electronystagmography (ENG) and the excitability of the vestibular sensory epithelia was investigated by observing the activity of succinic dehydrogenase (SDH) and Na^+-K^+-ATpase. SDH was stained by the same method as described by Nachlas et al. [1957] and Na^+-K^+-ATPase was stained by the method of Mayahara et al. [1980].

Clinical Study
The characteristic differences between I-ny and P-ny were investigated by computer analysis of electronystagmographs with 80 patients having unilateral peripheral vestibular disorder. On the other hand, the equilibrium function of the patients was investigated by computer analysis of the results of stabilometry which was performed on the same day with ENG testing.

Results

Experimental Study

Physiological Examination. The administration of potassium ion into the perilymph caused a reversible nystagmus. All experimental animals showed nystagmus directed to the iontophoretic ear which appeared about 15 min after iontophoresis and lasted for about 5 min. After a latent interval of a few minutes, a second nystagmus was developed and increased in amplitude and frequency. At this time, the direction of the nystagmus turned to the unaffected ear. This nystagmus gradually decreased its amplitude but lasted for 6–24 h. Despite this severe vertiginous attack, nystagmus was no longer visible on the next day. We called the first and the second nystagmus irritative and paralytic, respectively.

Histochemical Examination. In the irritative phase, the surface preparation of the crista ampullaris showed the more intensive activity of SDH and Na^+-K^+-ATPase in the iontophoretic ear than that in the unaffected ear. Electron microscopic observation detected that the intensive activity of Na^+-K^+-ATPase was mainly associated with the synaptic area between vestibular sensory cells and the nerve endings [Hozawa et al., 1986]. During the first 10 min or more in the paralytic phase, the same tendency could be observed. But in the later stage, the activity of SDH and Na^+-K^+-ATPase was decreased in the iontophoretic side, while that of the control side showed almost the same activity throughout this experiment. In spite of the decreased enzyme activity, no morphological change could be observed in the sensory cells nor in the nerve fibers.

Clinical Study

The mean values of each parameter of nystagmus is shown in table I. From computer analysis of ENG, the following results were obtained ($p < 0.05$): (1) I-ny appeared for a shorter duration than P-ny. P-ny was observed for a comparatively long time in the dark room. (2) I-ny had high frequencies, large amplitudes and fast slow-phase velocity, as compared with P-ny. (3) As to the interval variation, I-ny was regular as compared with P-ny at termination. (4) As to the amplitude variation, I-ny was larger than P-ny. (5) Most of the patients showing I-ny revealed the multi-eccentric body sway by analysis of the stabilograms. On the other hand, most of the patients with P-ny showed the lateral body sway. (6) Most of the patients with I-ny

Table I. Differing characteristics in irritative and paralytic nystagmus

	Irritative ny (n=40)			Paralytic ny (n=40)		
	ISP	SP	USP	ISP	SP	USP
Jerk number, per 20, s	16.3	15.2	20.2	18.9	15.1	13.7
Slow-phase velocity	3.4	4.4	4.0	4.0	2.7	2.7
Amplitude	2.3	2.5	2.7	1.3	1.7	1.4
Interval, ms	1,164	1,488	1,003	769	1,498	1,183
Interval variation, ms	442	647	542	651	651	744

ISP=Impaired side position; SP=sitting position; USP=unaffected side position.

complained of a turning sensation of surroundings, and the patients with P-ny had a swaying sensation of the body.

Discussion

The reversal of nystagmus direction was proved by many animal experiments and clinical reports concerning Ménière's attack [Arslan, 1963; Aschan, 1957; McClure et al., 1981; Meissner, 1981]. As a rule, ipsilateral and contralateral nystagmus are called irritative and paralytic, respectively. However, physiopathological conditions of the labyrinth to provoke the two types of nystagmus have not been clarified enough.

In our experiment, the change of vestibular cell excitability induced by the enzyme activity could correspond with the reversal of spontaneous nystagmus. That is, the vestibular sensory epithelia revealed the increased activity of SDH and Na^+-K^+-ATPase during ipsilateral I-ny and the decreased activity during contralateral P-ny.

There was some delay between the onset of P-ny and the beginning of the decrement of enzyme activity. This delay might be caused by the central regulatory mechanism for the disturbed tonus balance in the vestibular nucleus. On the other hand, our computer analysis revealed that the characteristic differences between I-ny and P-ny were observed not only in the direction but also in other parameters.

Although I-ny was observed for a comparatively short duration, it seemed to be provoked by strong and active energies of cell excitation of the unaffected side of the labyrinth. On the other hand, P-ny in the dark room had a comparatively long duration until it disappeared by the central compensation. P-ny seemed to be provoked by a relatively strong influence of the vestibular nucleus on the contralateral side, which was induced by the decrement of cell excitation of the impaired side of the labyrinth.

References

Arslan, M.: Origin of the nystagmus arising during and after ultrasonic destructive irradiation of the vestibular apparatus. Acta Oto-lar. suppl. 192, pp. 122–133 (1963).

Aschan, G.; Stahle, J.: Nystagmus in Ménière's disease during attacks. Acta oto-lar. 47: 189–201 (1957).

Hozawa, J.; Fukuoka, K.; Usami, S.; Kamimura, T.; Hozawa, K.: Experimental studies on mechanism of the Ménière's attack: investigation into vestibulo-cochlear response of the guinea pig induced by potassium ion. Auris, Nasus, Larynx, Tokyo 13: suppl. II, pp. 21–27 (1986).

Mayahara, H.; Fujimoto, K.; Ogawa, K.: A new one-step method for the cytochemical localization of ouabain-sensitive potassium-dependent p-nitrophenyl phosphate activity. Histochemistry 67: 125–138 (1980).

McClure, J.A.; Copp, J.C.; Lycett, P.: Recovery nystagmus in Ménière's disease. Laryngoscope 91: 1727–1737 (1981).

Meissner, R.: Behavior of the nystagmus in Meniere's attack. Archs Oto-Rhino-Lar. 233: 173–177 (1981).

Molinari, G.A.: Alterations of inner ear mechanisms resulting from application of sodium chloride to the round window membrane. Annls Oto-lar. 81: 315–322 (1972).

Nachlas, M.M.; Tsou, K.C.; Souza, E.; Cheng, C.S.; Seligman, A.M.: Cytochemical demonstration of succinic dehydrogenase by the use of a new p-nitrophenyl substituted ditetrasole. J. Histochem. Cytochem. 5: 420–436 (1957).

J. Hozawa, MD, Department of Otolaryngology, Hirosaki University School of Medicine, Zaifu Cho 5, Hirosaki 036 (Japan)

Adv. Oto-Rhino-Laryng., vol. 42, pp. 139–143 (Karger, Basel 1988)

Temporal Development of Experimental Hydrops in the Vestibular Organ

A.M. Meyer zum Gottesberge, A. Meyer zum Gottesberge

Research Laboratory for Experimental Otology and Physiology, ENT Department, University of Düsseldorf, Düsseldorf, FRG

Introduction

Calcium ions play a major role in the regulation of cell functions. Ca^{2+} homeostasis is governed by the way in which calcium entry into the cytosol is balanced by the pump mechanism which excludes calcium outward, because minor deviations may result in major functional alterations or even in irreversible cell damage [15]. The concentration of Ca^{2+} in the endolymph is 10–100 times lower than in the perilymph and the extracellular fluid [1, 2, 13]. Moreover, the concentration differs in the different inner ear compartments, such as in the cochlear duct, in the utricle/semicircular canal and in the endolymphatic sac [11]. The calcium equilibrium potential (E_{Ca}) according to the Nernst equation showed different main sources for calcium transport in each compartment and may therefore indicate a different distribution of the Ca^{2+} transporting mechanism.

The experimentally induced endolymphatic hydrops (EEH), by obliteration of the endolymphatic sac and duct, causes a disturbance of Ca^{2+} homeostasis in the inner ear which results in an increase of Ca^{2+} concentration in the endolymph as well as intracellularly [9].

The underlying mechanism of the pathophysiology of this important ion in EEH is not yet known. For better understanding it is important to explore the earliest point of time of the beginning of the hydrops. The question is whether only the mechanical obstruction alone causes hydrops or some 'unknown' chemical signal which acts as a modulator and influences the cells maintaining the ionic composition of the endolymph.

Whereas our previous measurements in EEH of guinea pigs were performed one year (endolymph) and 3 months (microprobe analysis) after obliteration [6, 12], the purpose of the present study is to follow retrogradely the time course of the development of the EEH to find the earliest response of the epithelial cells to the osmotic changes in regard to calcium. The secretory area of utricle and semicircular canal are assayed for structure changes using the light, electron microscope and microprobe analytical technique LAMMA (laser-induced mass microprobe analyzer) for intracellular ionic alteration.

Methods

In 20 pigmented guinea pigs the endolymphatic sac and duct were obliterated unilaterally. After a posterior fossa craniotomy the sac and duct were reached by an extradural approach and the duct drilled and occluded with bone wax ad modum Kimura [3]. Eight animals were studied electron-microscopically [6] after varying periods and until one month; 12 animals were studied after 1 h, 4 h, 1 day, 4 days, and 7 days after obliteration by intracellular ion measurement (using the LAMMA instrument). The method in detail is described elsewhere [14].

Results and Discussion

The secretory area of the utricular and ampullar wall consists of one layer of epithelial cells (dark and light cells). In a close relationship to these cells melanocytes are located. This morphological arrangement serves as an ideal model tissue to observe the response of the osmotic changes in the endolymph. The morphology and presumptive function of the dark cells are more documented [4] contrarily to the light cells which are species-dependent and irregularly distributed between the dark cells. Both cell types differ in ion content [5]. The dark cells contain much more potassium and magnesium, whereas the light cells contain more sodium and traces of calcium.

In the preliminary present study the alterations in the shape of the light cells were observed 1 h after surgical procedure. However, the cells on the control side showed similar reactions. After one day the cells on the control side had recovered while the volume of the light cells on the operated side continuously increased until 4–7 days when the maximum cellular alterations occurred (fig. 1). The LAMMA measurements determine a time-dependent increase of calcium content in the light cells during the first week correlated to the cellular alteration (fig. 2). The K/Na ratio of the cells did not change significantly in the dark cells with the exception in measurements obtained 1 h after obliteration when a little shift was observed.

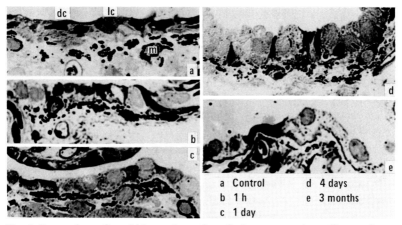

Fig. 1. Comparison of semithin sections of vestibular secretory layer (frozen, freeze-dried and tissue-embedded in Spurr's resin as prepared for LAMMA analysis) in different time schedules after obliteration of the endolymphatic sac and duct. dc = Dark cell; lc = light cell; m = melanocyte.

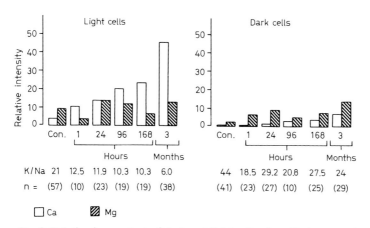

Fig. 2. Relative ion content of dark and light cells of vestibular organ in regard to calcium and magnesium. Con = control.

It seems that under pathological conditions the Ca^{2+} homeostasis of the light cells is disturbed. Accumulation may be due to an increase of calcium influx into the cells and/or to an insufficient outward pumping mechanism. Moreover, Ca^{2+} ATPase was described only in the basal infoldings of the dark cells; its presence in the light cells, however, is not mentioned by Yoshihara et al. [16]. It is possible that another ATPase-independent mechanism is involved in the Ca^{2+} homeostasis of these cells. The thickening of the basal membrane of the light cells gives morphological evidence for transmembrane transport. Furthermore, the large number of coated pits and vesicles on the luminal membrane indicates the possibility of a receptor binding site which may be involved in the Ca^{2+} transport. Finally, an enlarged endoplasmatic reticulum may play an active role in sequestering calcium [unpublished observation].

It is obvious that melanin is involved in Ca^{2+} homeostasis of the inner ear [6, 7]. Initially, one day after obliteration, an increase of total calcium in melanosomes was determined, followed by a cytosolic increase of the melanocytes with consequent cellular responses, such as organelle/cell motility, formation of new melanosomes (increased buffer capacity of calcium?), and endocytotic/exocytotic processes. This was described in detail elsewhere [8, 10].

References

1 Bosher, S.K.; Warren, R.L.: Very low calcium content of cochlear endolymph, an extracellular fluid. Nature 27: 377–378 (1978).

2 Ikeda, K.; Kusakari, J.; Takasaka, T.; Saito, Y.: The Ca^{2+} activity of cochlear endolymph of the guinea pig and the effect of inhibitors. Hearing Res. 26: 117–126 (1986).

3 Kimura, R.: Experimental blockage of the endolymphatic duct and its effect on the inner ear of guinea pig. A study on endolymphatic hydrops. Annls Oto-lar. 76: 664–687 (1967).

4 Kimura, R.S.: Distribution, structure, and function of dark cells in the vestibular labyrinth. Annls Oto-lar. 78: 542–559 (1969).

5 Meyer zum Gottesberge-Orsulakova, A.; Kaufmann, R.: Recent advances in laser microprobe mass analysis (LAMMA) of inner ear tissue. SEM I: 393–405 (1985).

6 Meyer zum Gottesberge-Orsulakova, A.M.; Kaufmann, R.: Is an imbalanced calcium-homeostasis responsible for the experimentally induced endolymphatic hydrps? Acta otolaryngol (Stockh) 102: 93–98 (1986).

7 Meyer zum Gottesberge-Orsulakova, A.: Melanin in the inner ear: micromorphological and microanalytical investigations. Acta histochem., suppl. XXXII: 245–253 (1986).

8 Meyer zum Gottesberge, A.M.: Microanalytical investigations of the inner ear, uveal tract and retinal pigment epithelium melanin. Adv. Biosci. 62: 435–443 (1987).

9 Meyer zum Gottesberge, A.M.; Ninoyu, O.: A new aspect in pathogenesis of experimental hydrops: role of calcium. Aviat. Space Environ. Med. 58: suppl. A, pp. 240–246 (1987).

10 Meyer zum Gottesberge, A.M.: Modulation of melanocytes during experimentally induced endolymphatic hydrops. Acta histochem. (1987).

11 Ninoyu, O.; Meyer zum Gottesberge, A.M.: Ca^{++} activity in the endolymphatic space. Archs Oto-Rhino-Lar. *243:* 141–142 (1986).

12 Ninoyu, O.; Meyer zum Gottesberge, A.M.: Changes in Ca^{++} activity and DC potential in experimentally induced endolymphatic hydrops. Archs Oto-Rhino-Lar. *243:* 106–107 (1986).

13 Ninoyu, O.; Meyer zum Gottesberge, A.M.: Calcium transport in the endolymphatic space of cochlea and vestibular organ. Acta oto-lar. *102:* 222–227 (1986).

14 Orsulakova, A.; Morgenstern, C.; Kaufmann, R.; D'Haese, M.: The laser microprobe mass analysis technique in the studies of inner ear. SEM *IV:* 1763–1766 (1982).

15 Peters, T.: Calcium in physiological and pathological cell function. Eur. Neurol. *25:* suppl. 1, pp. 27–44 (1986).

16 Yoshihara, T.; Igarashi, M.; Usami, S.; Kanda, T.: Cytochemical studies of Ca^{++}-ATpase activity in the vestibular epithelia of the guinea pig. Archs Oto-Rhino-Lar. *243:* 417–423 (1987).

A.M. Meyer zum Gottesberge, PhD, Research Laboratory for Experimental Otology and Physiology, ENT-Department, University of Düsseldorf, Düsseldorf (FRG)

Adv. Oto-Rhino-Laryng., vol. 42, pp. 144–147 (Karger, Basel 1988)

Hearing in Patients with Ménière's Disease after Exposure to Low Ambient Pressure and after Ingestion of Glycerol and Urea

H.C. Larsen, C. Angelborg, I. Klockhoff, J. Stahle

ENT Department, Akademiska Sjukhuset, Uppsala University, Uppsala, Sweden

Introduction

In patients with Ménière's disease hearing can be transiently improved by hyperosmotic diuretics [Klockhoff and Lindblom, 1967; Angelborg et al., 1977, 1981; Larsen et al., 1984]. Also changes of the ambient pressure have been reported to have a positive effect on hearing [Densert et al., 1975; Tjernström et al., 1980; Densert and Densert, 1982]. The present study was performed to compare the effects of underpressure, on the one hand, and the effect of hyperosmotic diuretics, on the other, on the same patients with Ménière's disease.

Methods and Material

In 42 volunteering patients with Ménière's disease, all with the classical triad of symptoms, pure tone and speech audiometry was performed immediately before and after lowering of ambient pressure in a pressure chamber. Twenty-eight of these patients were women and 14 men, and the mean age was 53 ± 12 years. The duration of the disease varied between 1 and 18 years.

The underpressure exposure was performed in a low-pressure chamber with space for 6 persons. The patients were placed in a sitting position during the test. In 30 patients the pressure was lowered by 5 kPa below atmospheric pressure for 5 min and later to 10 kPa for 5 min. It took about 1 min to lower the pressure within the chamber from atmospheric pressure to 10 kPa and 8 s to bring the pressure back to normal again.

In 12 patients the pressure was lowered to 10 kPa for 10 min on three occasions. Two days later these patients underwent either of two hyperosmotic tests. On an empty stomach 6 patients were given 1.5 g glycerol per kilogram body weight and 6 others got 0.6 g urea per kilogram body weight. Pure tone and speech audiometry were performed before and 2 h after the administration of the hyperosmotic solutions.

The results of the audiometric tests were judged according to criteria previously set for a positive glycerol test; a mean pure-tone threshold improvement of at least 10 dB in 2 adjacent octave bands and/or an improvement of the speech audiometry of at least 10%.

Results

Positive audiometric tests, i.e. a significant reduction of hearing loss, were achieved in 12 of the 42 (29%) patients exposed to underpressure. Eighteen patients reported a reduction of tinnitus or fullness in the ear, 5 patients reported a long-lasting improvement concerning vertigo whereas 3 reported that their vertigo became worse. In 2 cases audiometric tests were repeated 2 days after the underpressure exposure but the hearing improvement registrated earlier was no longer present.

Of the 12 patients exposed to both underpressure and hyperosmotic testing only 3 (25%) showed positive responses to both tests. Six (50%) patients presented a positive hearing test only after hyperosmotic testing and 5 (41%) to the underpressure procedure only. Side effects due to the pressure changes were limited to slight dizziness during the rise in pressure, and a feeling of transient pressure in the ear.

Discussion

As described earlier by Densert et al. [1975], the exposure of Ménière patients to changes of ambient pressure may induce an improvement of their hearing. The vertiginous symptoms were also reduced in some patients. The positive effects on the symptoms in Ménière's disease did not remain for longer periods. Thus, the lowering of ambient pressure cannot be regarded as a new way of treating Ménière's disease. A positive response to underpressure can only for the time being be regarded as another way of indicating endolymphatic hydrops.

The fact that only 29% of the patients treated with 5 and 10 kPa underpressure for 10 min had an improvement in audiogram, and that 41% were improved after 10 min three times at 10 kPa, indicates that the pressure effect depends both on time and size of pressure. The findings of 50% positive hyperosmotic tests are in accordance with earlier reports [Klockhoff and Lindblom, 1967; Angelborg et al., 1977], suggesting that the previous under-pressure test in reality did not interfere.

In the 12 patients tested with both underpressure and either glycerol or urea, the correlation between the effects on hearing was low; only 3 patients were positive to both alternatives. This may be interpreted as the hearing improvement being achieved in different ways by hyperosmosis and changes of ambient pressure. In the low-pressure test Densert et al. [1975] have sug-gested that pressure changes affect the inner ear either by improving the inner ear blood flow or by means of reopening of a blocked endolymphatic duct.

The hyperosmotic tests, on the other hand, are supposed to act by means of extraction of fluid from the inner ear [Klockhoff and Lindblom, 1967; Angelborg et al., 1977], thereby reducing the endolymphatic hydrops. Direct support for the latter hypothesis is found in animal experiments showing that hyperosmotic solutions lower the inner ear pressure [Angelborg and Ågerup 1975; Carlborg and Farmer, 1983].

The inner ear blood flow may also be of importance for hearing loss and hearing fluctuations in Ménière's disease [Angelborg et al., 1981]. However, it is thought to be of minor importance in inducing the hearing improve-ments found in hyperosmotic tests [Larsen et al., 1981]. In tests using changes of ambient pressure, on the other hand, the blood flow may be of greater importance. This question will be further investigated.

References

Angelborg, C.; Ågerup, B.: Glycerol effects on the perilymphatic and cerebrospinal pressure. Acta oto-lar. *79:* 81 (1975).

Angelborg, C.; Klockhoff, I.; Larsen, H.C.; Stahle, J.: Hyperosmotic solutions and hearing in Ménière's disease. Am. J. Otol. *3:* 200 (1981).

Angelborg, C.; Klockhoff, I.; Stahle, J.: Urea and hearing in patients with Ménière's disease. Scand. Audiol. *6:* 143 (1977).

Carlborg, B.; Farmer, J.C.: Effects of hyperosmolar solutions on labyrinth pressures. Ann. Otol. Rhinol. Lar. *92:* 2 (1983).

Densert, B.; Densert, O.: Overpressure in treatment of Ménière's disease. Laryngoscope *92:* 1285 (1982).

Densert, O.; Ingelstedt, A.; Ivarsson, A.; Pedersen, K.: Immediate restoration of basal sensorineural hearing (Mb Ménière) using a pressure chamber. Acta oto-lar. *80:* 80 (1975).

Klockhoff, I.; Lindblom, U.: Glycerol test in Ménière's disease. Acta oto-lar., suppl. 224, p. 449 (1967).

Larsen, H.C.; Angelborg, C.; Hultcrantz, E.: Cochlear blood flow related to hyperosmotic solutions. Archs Oto-Rhino-Lar. *234:* 145 (1981).
Larsen, H.C.; Angelborg, C.; Klockhoff, I.; Stahle, J.: The effect of isosorbid and urea on H.C. Larsen, MD, ENT-Department, Akademiska Sjukhuset, Uppsala University, S–7585 Uppsala (Sweden)
Tjernström, Ö.; Casselbrant, M.; Harris, S.; Ivarsson, A.: Current status of pressure chamber treatment. Otolaryngol. Clin. North Am. *4:* 723 (1980).

H.C. Larsen, MD, ENT-Department, Akademiska Sjukhuset, Uppsala University, S–7585 Uppsala (Sweden)

Adv. Oto-Rhino-Laryng., vol. 42, pp. 148–152 (Karger, Basel 1988)

Perilymphatic Fistulae: A Single-Blind Clinical Histopathologic Study[1]

Robert I. Kohut, Raul Hinojosa, Jai H. Ryu

Section on Otolaryngology, Department of Surgery, Bowman Gray School of Medicine, Wake Forest University, Winston-Salem, N.C., and Section on Otolaryngology, University of Chicago Medical Center, Chicago, Ill., USA

Robert Barany made comments concerning fistulae symptoms at Ruttin's [1] 1909 presentation concerning fistulae in the oval window. Barany's thoughts at that time allowed the conclusion that the fistula symptom could be caused by an abnormally mobile stapes. Six years later Ruttin's data concerning the fistula symptom without histologic findings of a fistula tended to support Barany's conclusions [2].

Distinctly this seemed to be a strong possibility. Even Leidler [3] and McKenzie [4] were criticized when at surgery they could not identify any evidence for fistulae in patients in whom they had made this diagnosis. They operated without the aid of optical magnification.

Holmgren, in 1924, during an operation on the promontory for otosclerosis, was the first to observe a flow of clear fluid from the stapes area. He was using the operating microscope that he had developed. Twenty years later, during Wilson's [5] paper on the fissula ante fenestram, Holmgren recalled his unexplained observation and concluded that this fenestra was the source of the fluid that he had observed.

In the last 20 years, following observations of post-stapedectomy fistulae, clinical and surgical observations have been recorded concerning spontaneous fistulae of the oval and round windows of the labyrinthine capsule [6].

Based on clinical and surgical observations, we recently described [7] histologic criteria which demonstrate patency between the middle ear and the inner surface of the labyrinthine capsule by way of the fissula ante fenestram and the round window fissure. Using normal controls and based

[1] This study is funded in part by the Research Fund of the American Otological Society and National Institutes of Health Grant NS 22042.

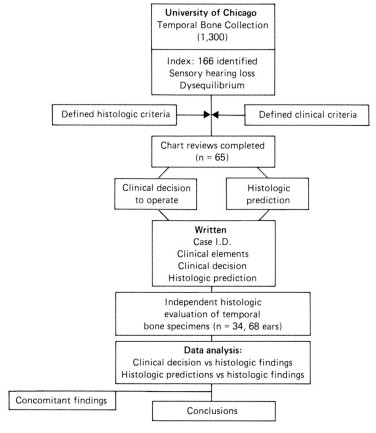

Fig. 1. Paradigm for study.

on this histologic evidence, we predicted, prior to chart review, the clinical elements of hearing loss and/or vertigo that were present during life.

The purpose of this paper is to describe a single-blind clinical histopathologic study concerning perilymphatic fistulae. The experimental paradigm is illustrated in figure 1. From the index of a collection of 1,300 temporal bones, 166 cases were identified that had sensory hearing loss and/or vertigo. Using predefined clinical criteria (table I) for the diagnosis of a perilymphatic leak, the charts were independently reviewed by one of the authors (R.K.) and a diagnosis was made without review of the histologic material. (The diagnosis had two parts: a hypothetical decision to explore the ear and/or a prediction

Table I. Identified clinical criteria. Cases without evidence for granulomatous, inflammatory, or neoplastic disorders.

Sensory hearing loss	Dysequilibrium (vertigo)
SXS	
(1) Sudden	(1) constant imbalance when upright
(2) Rapidly progressive	(2) postural vertigo (with transient positional nystagmus)
(3) Fluctuating with progressive loss	(3) Tullio phenomenon
Signs	
Sensory loss using audiometric tuning fork findings	
	(1) Hennebert's sign (fistula test)
	(2) Hennebert's symptom
	(3) positional nystagmus (with transitional postural vertigo)
	(4) unsteady gait or positive Romberg (Mann)

of histologic patency. These were identified and recorded as independent variables.) The experiment's design required that a decision had to be made even if the available data were only partially adequate. One other author (R.H.), using predefined histologic criteria [7], made an independent histologic diagnosis of patency of the fissula and/or fissure without knowledge of the clinical prediction of patency.

Results

Of the 166 cases identified from the temporal bone index collection, 65 chart reviews have been completed and the clinical decisions recorded. Of these 65 cases, 34 (68 ears) were available for histologic review. The clinical and histopathologic findings of these 34 cases (68 ears) are the data of this preliminary report. Of the 34 cases, 22 had hearing loss only, one had vertigo only, and 11 had hearing loss and vertigo.

Clinical Predictions. There were 11 cases (22 ears) that would have been hypothetically explored surgically. In 10 of these cases, 19 ears were histologically patent using the defined criteria (86% accuracy), 18 cases (36 ears) would not have been hypothetically explored surgically. In one of these nonexplored cases (2 ears), patency was present (94% accuracy); 5 cases had totally inadequate information with which to make a clinical decision. The histologic predictions had a similar degree of accuracy.

Bilateral patency (both ears) was present in 90% of the cases of the 19 ears with patency; 6 were of the oval window, 5 of the round window, and 8 of both the oval and round window. Of the 14 oval window areas having patency of the fissula, 6 also had ante mortem microfissures allowing for communication between the inner and middle ear. One of these 6 also had a histologically patent fossula post fenestram.

Concomitant (preliminary) histologic findings which were present in some cases included: (1) labyrinthine hydrops; (2) cochlear hair cell loss; (3) spiral ganglion cell loss; (4) vestibular labyrinthine compression, and (5) calcium deposits in the round window fissure.

Conclusions

(1) Single-blind clinical histopathologic studies can be performed. (2) The clinical criteria identified are predictors of the patency of the fissula ante fenestram and/or the round window fissure. (3) No histologic evidence for round window membrane rupture was observed. (4) The clinical entity 'perilymphatic leaks' is likely due to patency of the fissula ante fenestram and/or the round window fissure. (5) Patencies (fistulas) are commonly bilateral. (6) A microfracture or a patent fossula post fenestram may be a source of perilymph leakage to the middle ear. (7) This study can be independently repeated by others using the same materials.

References

1   Ruttin, E.: Fistel im ovalen Fenster. Mschr. Ohrenheilk. *10:* 787 (1909).
2   Ruttin, E.: Über Fistelsymptom ohne Fistel. Verh. Ges. dt. Hals-Nas.-Ohrenärzte *8:* 286 (1921).
3   Leidler, R.: Beitrag zur Pathologie des Bogengangsapparates. Z. Ohrenheilk. *56:* 328 (1908).
4   McKenzie, D.: The clinical value of the labyrinthine nystagmus test (analysis of forty-two cases). J. Lar. Otol. *24:* 646 (1909).
5   Wilson, J.G.: Fissula ante fenestram and adjacent tissue in the human otic capsule. Acta oto-lar. *22:* 382–389 (1935).

6   Mattox, D.: Perilymph fistulas; in Cummings, Fredrickson, Harker, Krause, Schuller, Otolaryngology—head and neck surgery (Mosby, St. Louis 1986).
7   Kohut, R.I.; Hinojosa, R.; Budetti, J.A.: Perilymphatic fistula: a histopathologic study. Ann. Otol. Rhinol. Lar. *95:* 466–471 (1986).

Robert I. Kohut, MD, FACS, Section Otolaryngology, Department of Surgery, Bowman Gray School of Medicine, Winston-Salem, NC 27103 (USA)

Adv. Oto-Rhino-Laryng., vol. 42, pp. 153–156 (Karger, Basel 1988)

Otolithic Tullio Phenomenon Typically Presents as Paroxysmal Ocular Tilt Reaction

T. Brandt, M. Dieterich, W. Fries

Neurologische Universitätsklinik, Klinikum Grosshadern, München, FRG

Sound induced vestibular symptoms such as vertigo, nystagmus, oscillopsia, and postural imbalance in patients with perilymphatic fistulas are commonly known as the Tullio phenomenon [Tullio, 1929]. Evidence is presented — based on otoneurological examination of a recent patient as well as re-evaluation of cases described in literature — that an *otolithic Tullio phenomenon* due to a hypermobile stapes footplate typically manifests with the pattern of sound induced paroxysms of ocular tilt reaction (OTR).

The patient, a professional horn player, complained about distressing attacks of vertical-oblique and rotatory oscillopsia (apparent counterclockwise tilt of the visual scene) as well as postural imbalance (fall towards the right and backward) elicited by loud sounds particularly when applied to the left ear with a maximum at a frequency of 480 $\pm$ 20 Hz. Uttering vowels, playing the horn or blowing the nose caused similar symptoms of varying severity.

Objectively simultaneous paroxysms of eye-head synkinesis (OTR) could be observed with the triad of skew deviation (ipsilateral over contralateral hypertropia), ocular torsion (counterclockwise), and head tilt (ipsilateral ear up). Electronystagmographic recordings as well as special video analysis (time resolution: 1,000 images/s) revealed a latency for the eye movements of 22 ms with an initial rapid and phasic rotatory-upward deviation (4°) which was followed by a smaller tonic effect as long as sound stimulation lasted (fig. 1). Skew deviation was caused by a disconjugate larger deviation of the ipsilateral eye. With repetitive sound stimulation habituation of the phasic component of eye movements occurred. A surprisingly short latency vestibulospinal reflex was recorded electromyographically [Fries et al., 1989] with an EMG response after 47 ms in the tibialis anterior muscle and after 52 ms in the gastrocnemius muscle at upright stance (fig. 2).

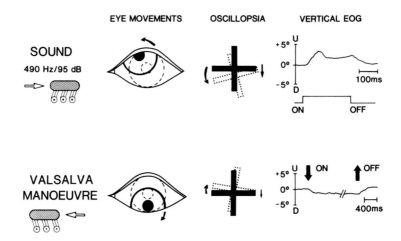

Fig. 1. Tullio phenomenon of sound-induced eye movements due to a hypermobile stapes footplate left ear. The sound causes a rapid and phasic eye movement oblique upward with incyclotropia and concomitant oscillopsia with counterclockwise tilt of the visual scene. A smaller tonic deviation of the eyes maintains as long as the sound lasts (top). Increasing intracranial pressure by Valsalva maneuver causes (smaller) slow and tonic eye movements and oscillopsia opposite in direction to the Tullio phenomenon (bottom). The opposite directions of eye movements may reflect push or pull stimulation of the otoliths.

A considerable postural perturbation was measured by means of a Kistler platform with the shortest latency of 80 ms and a preferred body sway direction from right-backward to left-forward.

Increasing intracranial pressure by Valsalva maneuver evoked slow tonic eye movements and oscillopsia opposite in direction to those of the Tullio phenomenon (fig. 1). Surgical exploration of the middle ear (Dr. Scherer, ENT Department) revealed a subluxated stapes footplate with the hypertrophic stapedius muscle causing pathological large amplitude movements during the stapedius reflex. This explains why the Tullio phenomenon could be evoked (but with weaker effects) by sound stimulation of the right ear.

Obviously, otolithic stimulation is the cause of the described symptoms. OTR first delineated by Westheimer and Blair in 1975 represents a fundamental pattern of coordinated eye-head motion in roll based upon utricular/saccular input. It has been described for a partial lesion of the utricle following stapedectomy [Halmagyi et al., 1980] and for lesions of the graviceptive pathways to rostral midbrain tegmentum [Brandt and Diete-

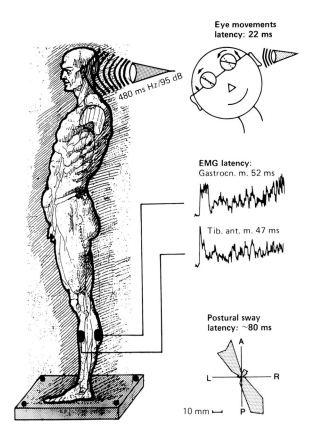

Fig. 2. The complete Tullio phenomenon in the patient is characterized by an OTR (top) and a sound-induced increased body sway predominantly from right-backward to left-forward (bottom). Latencies of disconjugated eye movements were 22 ms; latencies for the vestibulospinal reflex (mediated by otolithic stimulation) was as short as 47 ms (tib. ant. m.) whereas measurable postural sway had a minimal latency of 80 ms.

rich, 1987]. In the Tullio phenomenon hypermetric pumping movements of the stapes appear the most likely cause for inadequate stimulation of the adjacent otoliths. The opposite directions of the eye movements induced either by sound or Valsalva maneuver would then reflect a push and pull of the otoliths, respectively.

Thus, an otolithic type can be differentiated within the heterogeneous group of Tullio phenomena which must be distinguished from a semicircular canal (nystagmus) type, e.g. due to window rupture. The well-documented earlier case descriptions by Deecke et al. [1981] and by Vogel et al. [1986] most probably meant the same disease since they include features of OTR, although the syndrome was termed differently. These authors already discussed a possible otolithic mechanism, however, without a surgical proof of the site of the fistula.

References

Brandt, T.; Dieterich, M.: Pathological eye-head coordination in roll: tonic ocular tilt reaction in mesencephalic and medullary lesions. Brain *110:* 649–666 (1987).

Deecke, L.; Mergner, T.; Plester, D.: Tullio phenomenon with torsion of the eyes and subjective tilt of the visual surround. Ann. N.Y. Acad. Sci. *374:* 650–655 (1981).

Fries, W.; Dieterich, M.; Brandt, T.: Vestibulo-spinal reflexes in man: otolithic contributions to postural mechanisms. Exp. Brain Res. (1989).

Halmagyi, G.M.; Gresty, M.A.; Gibson, W.P.R.: Ocular tilt reaction with peripheral vestibular lesions. Ann. Neurol. *6:* 80–83 (1980).

Tullio, P.: Sulla funzione delle varie partie dell'orecchio interno (German translation: Das Ohr und die Entstehung von Sprache und Schrift) (Urban & Schwarzenberg, Berlin 1929).

Vogel, P.; Tackmann, W.; Schmidt, F.-J.: Observations on the Tullio phenomenon. J. Neurol. *233:* 136–139 (1986).

Westheimer, G.; Blair, S.M.: The ocular tilt reaction — a brainstem ocular motor routine. Investve Ophth. *14:* 833–839 (1975).

Prof. Dr. Thomas Brandt, Neurologische Universitätsklinik,Klinikum Grosshadern, Marchioninistrasse 15, 8000 München 70 (FRG)

Adv. Oto-Rhino-Laryng., vol. 42, pp. 157–161 (Karger, Basel 1988)

Vestibular Neuritis —
A Horizontal Semicircular Canal Paresis?

W. Büchele, T. Brandt

Neurologische Universitätsklinik, Klinikum Grosshadern, München, FRG

Schuknecht and Kitamura [1981] presented histological evidence that the well-known clinical entity of an acute unilateral loss of peripheral vestibular function is due to vestibular nerve site viral inflammation rather than a vascular ischemia, thus confirming that the term *vestibular neuritis (VN)* is definitely correct. In the recent review of Baloh et al. [1987] on 240 cases of *benign paroxysmal positioning vertigo (BPPV)* it is stated that 15% are the sequelae of viral neurolabyrinthitis. The coincidence of both a complete VN and BPPV in the same individuum in the same ear at the same time seems impossible since it implicates function and loss of function of one labyrinthine structure at the same time. The repeated clinical observation of this apparently paradoxical coincidence led us to the following considerations.

According to Schuknecht's hypothesis of cupulolithiasis [Schuknecht, 1969; Schuknecht and Ruby, 1973] BPPV requires a preserved function of the ipsilateral posterior semicircular canal and its ampullary nerve. This is supported by Gacek [1984] who was able to successfully heal intractable cases by selective sectioning of the posterior ampullary nerve. Consequently — with respect to VN — a question arises whether in the cases of VN plus BPPV only part of the vestibular nerve, i.e. the superior division, is defective (fig. 2c) whereas the inferior part is spared.

We found that 12% of a total of 104 patients with clinically diagnosed unilateral BPPV reported a prior episode of continuous vertigo compatible with VN days to years previously. In all of them thermic irrigation revealed an ipsilateral under- (60%) or unresponsiveness (40%) and in some there was still a spontaneous nystagmus present with its fast phase beating towards the unaffected ear (fig. 1). On the other hand, 6 out of 76 patients who were

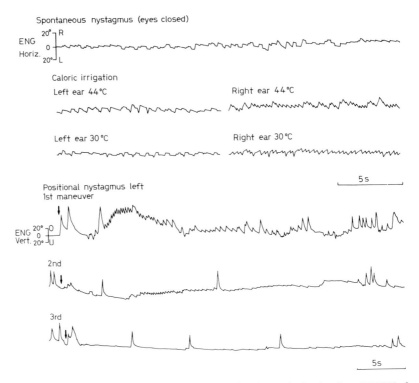

Spontaneous nystagmus (eyes closed)

Caloric irrigation
Left ear 44 °C   Right ear 44 °C

Left ear 30 °C   Right ear 30 °C

Positional nystagmus left
1st maneuver

2nd

3rd

Fig. 1. Original recordings of a patient (H.S., male, 48 years) who developed BPPV of the left ear 4 weeks after VN in the same ear. There is still a spontaneous nystagmus present to the right; thermic irrigation reveals unresponsiveness of the horizontal canal (top). Typical BPPV (vertical trace) in the same patient with fatigue during the third positioning maneuver (bottom).

observed clinically following a complete VN after a varying latency of 4–8 weeks reported a spontaneous change in vertigo character with the typical features of an ipsilateral BPPV even though thermic irrigation still showed no response on the affected side. Physical therapy by systematically repeated positioning maneuvers [Brandt and Daroff, 1980] cured only two-thirds of these cases compared to a 90% efficacy in a group of patients without concurrent VN. One female (aged 25 years) who did not respond to physical treatment at all was finally successfully operated on (Dr. H. Scherer, ENT Department) by selective sectioning of the posterior ampullary nerve.

Since its first description, Schuknecht's [1969] theory of cupulolithiasis has been the object of critical debates. Schmidt [1985] stated that the typical

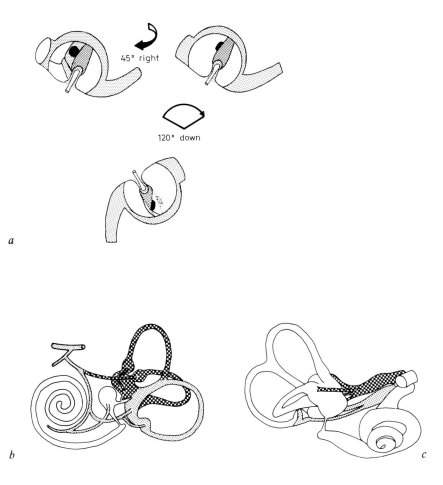

a

b   *c*

Fig. 2. a Schematic drawing of cupulolithiasis with ampullofugal deflection of the cupula by a provocative head positioning maneuver when the posterior canal is rapidly moved in the specific plane of stimulation. *b* Theoretical vascular explanation of the coincidence of BPPV and VN when the anterior vestibular artery is affected only sparing the posterior branch which supplies the posterior canal. *c* Possible viral etiology of VN affecting parts of the nerve, in particular horizontal ampullary nerve, but sparing the inferior division the function of which is necessary for the occurrence of BPPV in the same ear.

nystagmus pattern in BPPV must be due to an ampullofugal rather than an ampullopetal deflection of the cupula according to the animal experiments by Cohen [1974]. He did not believe in cupulolithiasis, but explained BPPV as the consequence of impaired utricular function which causes an overexcitability of the normal postrotatory response of the posterior canal. As shown in figure 2a, however, the necessity of ampullofugal deflection of the cupula does not exclude the mechanism of cupulolithiasis. The symptoms of BPPV are compatible with the cupulogram of an ampullofugal stimulation of the posterior canal of the undermost ear when the 'heavy cupula' creates an overexcitability of the particular canal to angular accelerations in the specific plane.

The earlier hypothesis of Lindsay and Hemenway [1956], on the other hand, would allow a convincing explanation for the coincidence of VN and BPPV on the basis of a vascular pathogenesis. If an ischemic event only involves the anterior vestibular artery this would cause a contraversive horizontal nystagmus in the acute stage with ipsilateral unresponsiveness to thermic irrigation of the horizontal canal and could also promote cupulolithiasis of otoconia by ischemic degeneration of the utricular macula. Basophilic material attached to the cupula of the posterior canal was in fact found by Schuknecht and Ruby [1973] in their rare proven cases of BPPV with cupulolithiasis. Since the cupula of the posterior canal, like the cochlear duct and part of the sacculus, get their blood supply from another arterial branch, their function would be preserved — a physiological precondition for the occurrence of BPPV (fig. 2b).

Schuknecht and Kitamura [1981] convincingly disproved the vascular etiology of VN and even tried to declare Lindsay and Hemenway's cases as being of the same viral etiology. Thus, one must then assume that at least in the patients with VN and concurrent BPPV only the superior division of the vestibular nerve, which travels separately and has its own ganglion, is affected (fig. 2c). This leaves us with the question of why and how under these conditions the mechanical process of cupulolithiasis occurs so frequently. Further studies are required in patients with combined VN and BPPV in order to prove preserved function of the posterior canal while the horizontal canal is paretic and to compare the results with those of 'normal' BPPV and VN patients.

It is our current concept that vestibular neuritis with the diagnostic hallmark of ipsilateral thermic hyporesponsiveness is a partial rather than a complete vestibular paresis with predominant involvement of the horizontal canal.

References

Baloh, R.W.; Honrubia, V.; Jacobson, K.: Benign positional vertigo: clinical and oculographic features in 240 cases. Neurology *37:* 371–378 (1987).

Brandt, T.; Daroff, R.B.: Physical therapy for benign paroxysmal positional vertigo. Archs Otolar. *106:* 484–485 (1980).

Cohen, B.: The vestibulo-ocular reflex arc; in Kornhuber, Handbook of sensory physiology, VI/1, pp. 477–540 (Springer, Berlin 1974).

Gacek, R.R.: Cupulolithiasis and posterior ampullary nerve transection. Ann. Otol. Rhinol. Lar. *93:* suppl. 112, pp. 25–29 (1984).

Lindsay, J.R.; Hemenway, W.G.: Postural vertigo due to unilateral sudden partial loss of vestibular function. Annls Oto-lar. *65:* 692–706 (1956).

Schmidt, C.L.: Zur Pathophysiologie des peripheren, paroxysmalen, benignen Lagerungsschwindels (BPPV). Lar. Rhinol. Otol. *64:* 146–155 (1985).

Schuknecht, H.F.: Cupulolithiasis. Archs Otolar. *90:* 113–129 (1969).

Schuknecht, H.F.; Kitamura, K.: Vestibular neuritis. Ann. Otol. Rhinol. Lar. *90:* suppl. 78, pp. 1–19 (1981)

Schuknecht, H.F.; Ruby, R.R.F.: Cupulolithiasis. Adv. Oto-Rhino-Laryng., vol. 20, pp. 434–443 (Karger, Basel 1973).

W. Büchele, MD, Neurologische Universitätsklinik, Klinikum Grosshadern, Marchioninistrasse 15, D-8000 München 70 (FRG)

Adv. Oto-Rhino-Laryng., vol. 42, pp. 162–171 (Karger, Basel 1988)

Inner Ear Damage Induced by Bacteria. Morphological and Behavioral Study

Yasuo Harada, Masaya Takumida, Nobuharu Tagashira, Yutaka Nagasawa, Mamoru Suzuki

Department of Otolaryngology, Hiroshima University, School of Medicine, Minamiku, Hiroshima, Japan

Introduction

Inner ear damage is induced by a variety of causes. These include ototoxic drugs, acoustic trauma and infection. It is also known that some kind of bacteria causes inner ear damage and dysequilibrium. The authors employed *Mycobacterium fortuitum* to induce inner ear damage. Morphological changes of the inner ear were studied in comparison with behavioral changes.

Materials and Method

CBA/jNCrj strain mice with normal Preyer's reflex were used. 0.2-ml solutions containing $7–8 \times 10^6$ of the live *M. fortuitum* or its extract was one shot injected into the tail vein of the mice.

Extracts from the *M. fortuitum* ATCC 6841 were prepared as follows: *M. fortuitum* was cultured on modified sorton medium at 37 °C for 14 days. Cultured bacteria were then concentrated and cracked by ultrasonic manipulation and were centrifuged at 100,000 g for 120 min. The resultant supernatant fluid was then filtered and used as the extract.

Behavioral Tests

The behavior of the animals was observed on the day of inoculation, 3 days, 1 week and 2 weeks after inoculation, following Sekiguchi's method. The observation items include: (1) general behavior and standing posture; (2) Preyer's reflex; (3) transversing a narrow path; (4) descending on rope; (5) negative geotaxis; (6) grasping a rod, and (7) swimming.

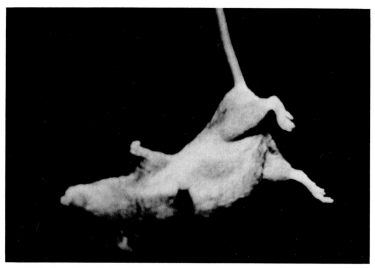

Fig. 1. M. fortuitum-induced spinning disease in the mouse 2 weeks after inoculation.

Morphological Observation

The inner ears were removed 3 days, 7 days, 2 weeks, 1 month and 3 months after inoculation of the live *M. fortuitum* and 2 weeks and 1 month after injection of the extract. Each animal was deeply anesthetized and was subjected to cardiac perfusion of 2.5% glutaraldehyde and 2% paraformaldehyde. The removed cochlea and the vestibular organs were postfixed in 2% OsO_4 and 2% tannic acid, and were dehydrated in ethanol. These specimens were then critical-point dried in CO_2 and were coated with platinum for scanning electron microscopic (SEM) observation. Some specimens were embedded in Epon after dehydration and ultrathin sections were processed for transmission electron microscopic (TEM) observation. SEM (Hitachi S800) and TEM (JEM 100CXII) were used for observation.

Results

Behavioral Tests

The Preyer's reflex disappeared 3 days after inoculation in 97.5% of the animals. 12.5 and 68.7% of the animals could not maintain normal posture 7 and 14 days after inoculation, respectively. Deterioration of transversing path, descending rope, negative geotaxis and grasping rod was noticed on 7 days (12.5–18.8% of the animals) and 14 days (62.5–75% of the animals). The animals could not swim on 7 days (31.2%) and 14 days (73.3%). When

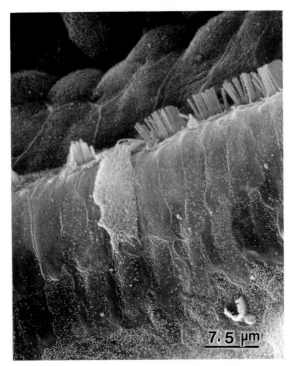

Fig. 2. The cochlea 3 days after inoculation. The stereocilia of the outer hair cell disappeared. Some of the remaining cilia show various degrees of change.

suspended by their tails, these mice rotated with such vigor that their bodies reached the horizontal plane (fig. 1).

Morphological Changes
Live *M. fortuitum* Injection Group
Changes of the Organ of Corti. Three days after inoculation, most of the outer hair cell (OHC) stereocilia were lost and some of the remaining cilia sustained various degrees of damage, such as fusion, disarray and complete loss. Changes of the inner hair cells (IHC) were less severe than those of the OHC. However, some of the IHC stereocilia were damaged or lost (fig. 2).

Two weeks after inoculation, the OHC stereocilia disappeared in all turns of the cochlea. The changes of the IHC stereocilia also developed. In the specimens taken between 2 and 4 weeks after the treatment, the damage of the IHC cilia extended toward the apical turn (fig. 3). One month after inoculation most of the IHC cilia disappeared in all turns.

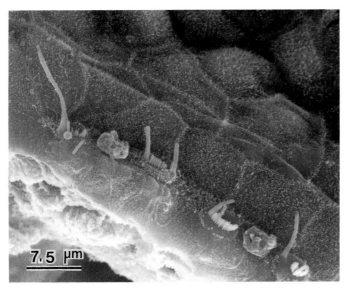

Fig. 3. The cochlea, 2 weeks after inoculation. The outer hair cell cilia have completely disappeared. The inner hair cells show ballooning and have giant or fused cilia.

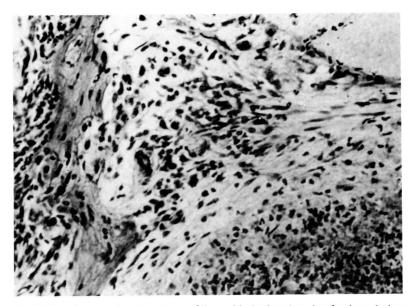

Fig. 4. The spiral ganglion (lower turn of the cochlea) taken 4 weeks after inoculation. Loss of the ganglion cell is obvious.

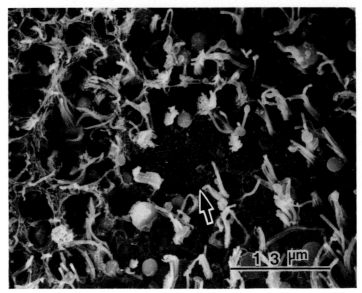

Fig. 5. The utricular macula, 2 weeks after inoculation. The damage of the cilia is severe in the striola portion (arrow).

Changes of the Spiral Ganglion. Three days after inoculation the spiral ganglion already showed some changes. The initial change was degeneration of the mitochondria. The damage progressed to change of the Golgi apparatus, swelling of the cisterns with vacuolization in the rough endoplasmic reticulum and degeneration of the myelin sheath. Later, the loss of the ganglion cell was obvious in all turns of the cochlea and the nerve fibers in the modiolus were also degenerated (fig. 4).

Changes of the Vestibular Organs. No change was observed until 7 days after inoculation. Two weeks later changes were noticed in the striola portion of the utricular macula (fig. 5). The change of the cilia includes disappearance, fusion and ballooning. Ballooning of the top of the cilia seems to be the most specific finding in the present study (fig. 6). TEM revealed sensory hair damage and protrusion of the sensory and the supporting cell surface (fig. 7). The change also involved both the saccular macula and crista ampullaris and was the most obvious in the striola portion and in the top of the crista. During 1–3 months after inoculation these lesions of the hair cell became more noticeable. Furthermore, the nerve fibers running in the neurovascular

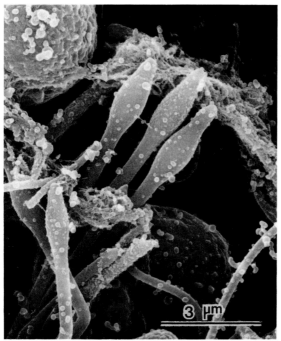

Fig. 6. The utricular macula, 2 weeks after inoculation, showing ballooning of the top of the cilia.

layer also showed morphological changes. Degeneration or loss of the intra-axonal mitochondria and vacuolization or dissociation of the myelin sheath were observed (fig. 8).

Changes of the Vestibular Ganglion. No change was observed until 7 days after inoculation. However, 2 weeks later the number of ganglion cells was reduced to about half of that of the control. The damage progressed further at 4 weeks after inoculation (fig. 9).

Extract Injection Group

No change was observed until 2 weeks after injection. One month later the OHC stereocilia were degenerated and disappeared in the lower turn (fig. 10). In contrast, only mild changes occurred in the vestibular organs. The pattern of the damage was similar to that observed in the live *M. fortuitum* inoculation.

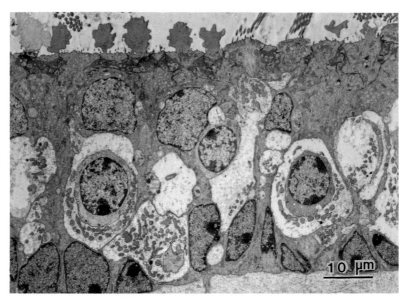

Fig. 7. The utricular macula, 2 weeks after inoculation. Both the sensory cell and the supporting cell are protruding toward the endolymphatic space.

Discussion

Inner ear damage can be induced by certain species of bacteria, such as *Pseudomonas pyocyanea*, Nocardia and Mycobacterium when they are injected intravenously [1]. Yet, little is known about the morphological changes produced by bacteria. The present study indicates that both *M. fortuitum* and its extract cause histological changes in the inner ear. In the organ of Corti, IHC and OHC cilia degenerated and disappeared within 3 days after inoculation. The pattern of these changes was similar to those induced by ototoxic drugs and acoustic trauma [2]. The OHC were generally more affected than the IHC, and the lower turn of the cochlea was more involved than was the upper turn. This difference in the severity of the damage found among the hair cells and the cochlear turns was also comparable to that induced by other causes. The vestibular changes occurred later than the cochlear changes. They were first noticed 2 weeks after inoculation. Disappearance, fusion and ballooning of the sensory hair were obvious in the striola portion of the macula and in the top of the crista ampullaris. These findings are also similar to those of ototoxic drugs [3].

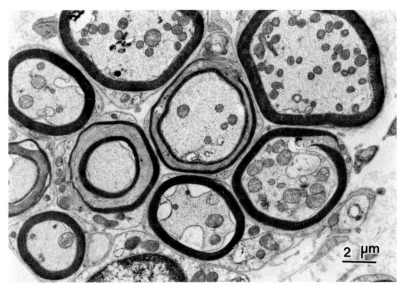

Fig. 8. The utricular nerve, 2 weeks after inoculation. The mitochondrial cristae are lost. The myelin sheath of the nerve fiber is dissociated and intra-axonal vacuolizations are obvious.

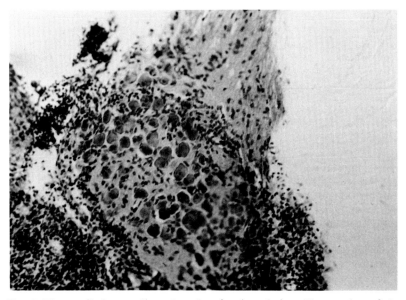

Fig. 9. The vestibular ganglion, 4 weeks after inoculation. The number of the ganglion cells reduced to half of the normal.

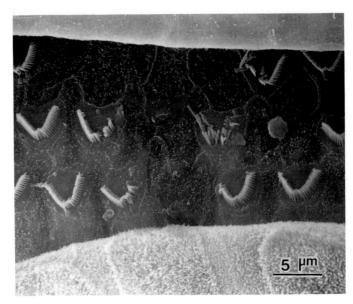

Fig. 10. The cochlea, one month after injection of the extract. Some outer hair cell stereocilia disappeared in the lower turn.

Concerning the mechanism of the bacterial inner ear damage, Nakai et al. [4] suggested that a Schwartzman reaction induced by the repeated injection of *E. coli* endotoxin lipopolysaccharide may also occur in other inner ear infections. Chemical changes in the inner ear fluid caused by infection might be another possible factor for inner ear disorder.

The present study has shown that pathological changes can also be induced by injections of bacterial extract. The damage caused by the extract were similar to those induced by the live bacteria. These injuries were dose-dependent and developed according to the survival time of the animals. Therefore, the inner ear disorders induced by *M. fortuitum* are possibly due to the effects of some component of its cell body.

A series of behavioral tests revealed that the onset of the equilibrium dysfunction basically coincides with that of the morphological changes. Therefore, the variety of dysequilibria could possibly be due to the extensive lesion in the inner ear. The test battery employed in this study may well serve as one of the parameters to evaluate vestibular function in the animals.

References

1   Gorrill, R.H.: Spinning disease of mice. J. Path. Bact. *71:* 353–358 (1956).
2   Harada, Y.: Atlas of the ear (MTP Press, Lancaster 1983).
3   Harada, Y.: The vestibular organs — morphology, physiology and pathology (Nishi-
    mura, Niigata 1984).
4   Nakai, Y.; Morimoto, A.; Chang, K.C.: Inner ear damage induced by bacterial
    endotoxin. Pract. Otol., Kyoto *71:* 559–571 (1978).

Y. Harada, MD, Department of Otolaryngology, Hiroshima University, School of
Medicine, 1-2-3 Kasumi, Minamiku, Hiroshima 734 (Japan)

Adv. Oto-Rhino-Laryng., vol. 42, pp. 172–176 (Karger, Basel 1988)

Histological Structures of Bilateral Acoustic Tumors

Ken Kitamura, Masahiro Sugimoto

Department of Otolaryngology, University of Tokyo, Tokyo, Japan

Introduction

Bilateral acoustic tumors, often felt to represent a central form of Recklinghausen's disease, show different clinical findings from unilateral tumors. There is less correlation between auditory findings and the tumor size of bilateral acoustic tumors than for unilateral tumors [1–3]. Auditory symptoms often do not occur in the case of large bilateral acoustic tumors. However, tumor expansion is more invasive than with unilateral tumors [2, 4]. The purpose of this study is to examine whether there are any different histological findings between bilateral and unilateral acoustic tumors.

Material and Methods

Tissue obtained from bilateral acoustic tumors from 12 patients (6 males, 6 females) was compared with tissue obtained from unilateral tumors from 6 patients (3 males, 3 females). In 9 of 12 patients with bilateral tumors, more than two symptoms of Recklinghausen's disease were present (café-au-lait spots, cutaneous tumors and some genetic component). The other 3 patients showed poor stigmata of Recklinghausen's disease. In addition, schwannomas of skin and spinal cord were demonstrated in these 3 patients. All specimens were obtained at surgery. Sections for light microscopy were stained with hematoxylin-eosin and Bodian. The sections were examined by the PAP (peroxidase-antiperoxidase) method, using rabbit antisera to S-100 protein (Dako Immunoglobulin Ltd., Denmark) in the primary, and anti-rabbit IgG swine serum in the secondary reaction. For electron microscopic study, specimens from 2 patients with bilateral acoustic tumors and 5 patients with unilateral acoustic tumors were fixed in 2% paraformaldehyde and 2% glutaraldehyde. They were postfixed with 2% osmium tetroxide, dehydrated through graded ethanol and embedded in Epon. Ultrathin sections were stained with uranyl acetate and lead citrate, and were examined with a Hitachi H 800 electron microscope.

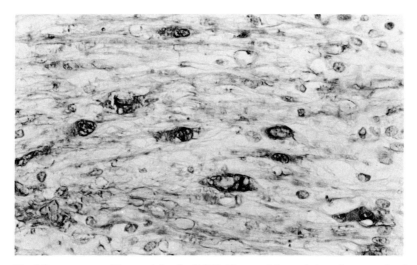

Fig. 1. Immunoperoxidase staining for S-100. Note positive staining of tumor cells of bilateral acoustic tumor. Counterstained with hematoxylin. ×300.

Findings

Both bilateral and unilateral acoustic tumors were composed of interwoven bundles of long spindle cells. An alignment of the nuclei known as palisading was demonstrated in 6 out of 12 patients with bilateral acoustic tumors and 3 out of 6 patients with unilateral acoustic tumors. No nerve fiber was demonstrated within the substance of either bilateral or unilateral acoustic tumors with a Bodian stain. Almost all tumor cells had diffuse immunoreactivity for S-100 protein in 11 patients with bilateral acoustic tumors, and all patients with unilateral acoustic tumors (fig. 1). Concentric whorls were demonstrated within the tumor in 2 patients with bilateral acoustic tumors. The cells composing the whorls were positive for S-100 protein.

Electron microscopic examination of bilateral and unilateral acoustic tumors revealed identical ultrastructural findings. Both of them were composed of tightly packed, long thin cells with complexly entangled processes separated at intervals by external lamina. Tumor cell nuclei were ovoid or rod-shaped. They generally had smooth surfaces; however, in some areas the nuclear surface was invaginated. Such invaginations contained cytoplasmic matter. Small numbers of mitochondria, scattered rough endoplasmic reticu-

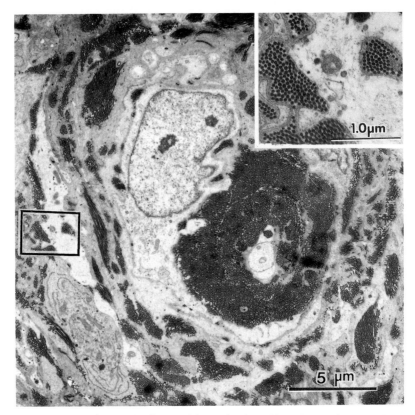

Fig. 2. Electron micrograph of a whorl formation in a bilateral acoustic tumor. Note numerous bundles of collagen and cells with complex processes. High power view of the bracketed area showing circumferentially oriented cell processes interdigitated with collagen bundles (inset).

lum and abundant microfilaments were seen in the cytoplasm. Long spacing collagen fibrils (Luse bodies) were numerous in the extracellular compartment. Two specimens of bilateral acoustic tumors demonstrated whorls which were composed of multiple concentric layers of thinned, markedly elongated cells and collagen bundles (fig. 2). The circumferentially oriented cell processes were complexly interdigitated with collagen bundles forming collagen pockets. An unmyelinated nerve fiber was observed in the center of the whorl. Typical fibroblasts with well-developed rough endoplasmic reticulum were rare in these specimens.

Discussion

There has been controversy with respect to the histology of bilateral acoustic tumors. Whereas some investigators [5, 6] suggested that bilateral acoustic tumors were neurofibromas, others [2, 4, 7] believed that both bilateral and unilateral acoustic tumors were schwannomas. In our study, patients with bilateral acoustic tumors were classified into two groups. The first group showed the stigmata of Recklinghausen's disease. The second might be referred to as the multiple neurilemmomas group [8]. Both groups demonstrated identical ultrastructural characteristics to unilateral acoustic tumors in this study. Whorls observed in bilateral acoustic tumors were similar to onion bulbs which were seen in various kinds of neuropathies, including hypertrophic neuropathy and peripheral neurofibromatosis [9, 10]. Although the presence of onion bulb formations was rare in neurinoma, it was recently demonstrated in the unilateral acoustic schwannoma [11]. All tumor cells of the 11 patients with bilateral acoustic tumors were strongly stained by S-100 protein immunohistochemistry. In schwannomas, all tumor cells were reported to be S-100-positive, and neurofibromas contained many S-100-protein-negative cells [12]. Thus, bilateral acoustic tumors were defined as schwannomas.

Although bilateral acoustic tumors could not be microscopically distinguished from unilateral ones, bilateral acoustic tumors were reported to be more invasive [2, 4]. On the contrary, hearing level and other neurological signs could be preserved more in patients with bilateral acoustic tumors than unilateral ones [1–3]. One of the possible proposals which could explain the discrepancy described above was the presence of remaining nerve fibers in the tumor substance [1, 2, 4]. In addition, Martuza and Ojemann [13] suggested that bilateral acoustic tumors were of multicellular origin and they surrounded cranial nerves as they enlarged. According to the biochemical method, Fabricant et al. [14] demonstrated that the antigenic activity of nerve growth factor was increased in sera from patients with bilateral acoustic tumors, whereas the functional activity was not increased. However, this did not seem to be conclusive evidence. In summary, we have postulated that bilateral acoustic tumors exhibit the histological features of schwannomas. Other histological or biochemical evidence which can determine the peculiar clinical findings of bilateral acoustic tumors has yet to be demonstrated.

References

1 Linthicum, F.H., Jr.: Unusual audiometric and histologic findings in bilateral acoustic neurinomas. Ann. Otol. Rhinol. Lar. *81:* 433–437 (1972).

2 Linthicum, F.H., Jr.; Brackmann, D.E.: Bilateral acoustic tumors. A diagnostic and surgical challenge. Archs Otolar. 106: 729–733 (1980).
3 Bess, F.H.; Josey, A.F.; Glasscock, M.E., III; Wilson, L.K.: Audiologic manifestations in bilateral acoustic tumors (von Recklinghausen's disease). J. Speech Hear. Disorders 49: 177–182 (1984).
4 Eckermeier, L.; Pirsig, W.; Mueller, D.: Histopathology of 30 nonoperated acoustic schwannomas. Archs Oto-Rhino-Lar. 222: 1–9 (1979).
5 Penfield, W.; Young, A.W.: The nature of von Recklinghausen's disease and the tumors associated with it. Archs neurol. Psychiat. 23: 320–344 (1930).
6 Gardner, W.J.; Turner, O.: Bilateral acoustic neurofibromas. Further clinical and pathologic data on hereditary deafness and Recklinghausen's disease. Archs neurol. Psychiat. 44: 76–99 (1940).
7 Nager, G.T.: Association of bilateral VIIIth nerve tumors with meningiomas in von Recklinghausen's disease. Laryngoscope 74: 1220–1261 (1964).
8 Shishiba, T.; Niimura, M.; Ohtsuka, F.; Tsuru, N.: Multiple cutaneous neurilemmomas as a skin manifestation of neurilemmomatosis. J. Am. Acad. Dermatol. 10: 744–754 (1984).
9 Dyck, P.J.: Inherited neuronal degeneration and atrophy affecting peripheral motor, sensory, and autonomic neurons; in Dyck, Thomas, Lambert, Bunge, Peripheral neuropathy, pp. 1600–1655 (Saunders, Philadelphia 1984).
10 Urich, H.: Pathology of tumors of cranial nerves, spinal nerve roots, and peripheral nerves; in Dyck, Thomas, Lambert, Bunge, Peripheral neuropathy, pp. 2253–2299 (Saunders, Philadelphia 1984).
11 Ylikoski, J.: Light and electron microscopic findings in a case of small acoustic schwannoma (associated with a schwannoma of the facial nerve). J. Lar. Otol. 100: 785–795 (1986).
12 Nakajima, T.; Kameya, T.; Watanabe, S.; Hirota, T.; Stato, Y.; Shimosato, Y.: An immunoperoxidase study of S-100 protein distribution in normal and neoplastic tissues. Am. J. surg. Pathol. 6: 715–727 (1982).
13 Martuza, R.L.; Ojemann, R.G.: Bilateral acoustic neuromas. Clinical aspects, pathogenesis and treatment. Neurosurgery 10: 1–12 (1982).
14 Fabricant, R.N.; Todaro, G.J.; Eldridge, R.: Increased levels of a nerve-growth-factor cross-reacting protein in central neurofibromatosis. Lancet i: 4–7 (1979).

Ken Kitamura, MD, Department of Otolaryngology, University of Tokyo,
7-3-1 Hongo, Bunkyo-ku, Tokyo 113 (Japan)

Adv. Oto-Rhino-Laryng., vol. 42, pp. 177–179 (Karger, Basel 1988)

Recovery of Resting Activity in the Ipsilateral Vestibular Nucleus Following Unilateral Labyrinthectomy: Noncommissural Influences

Paul F. Smith, Ian S. Curthoys

Vestibular Research Laboratory, Department of Psychology, University of Sydney, Sydney, NSW, Australia

The present study investigated: (1) the correlation between changes in the resting activity (RA) of neurons in the bilateral medial vestibular nuclei (MVN) and the compensation of spontaneous nystagmus (SN), up to one year following unilateral labyrinth deafferentation (ULD) in guinea pig; (2) the contribution of the Scarpa's ganglion neurons ipsilateral to the ULD and the brain stem vestibular commissures to the recovery of MVN RA.

Materials and Method

The experiments were performed on anesthetized guinea pigs (nembutal 30 mg/kg i.m. and innovar 0.75 ml/kg; 0.40 mg/kg fentanyl and 20 mg/kg droperidol i.m.), which were either bilaterally intact or at one of 3 stages of recovery from a unilateral surgical labyrinthectomy: 0–8, 52–60 h or 8–12 months postoperation (PO). The medial cerebellum was aspirated; action potentials from single MVN neurons were recorded extracellularly using glass microelectrodes; during neuronal recording, vision was occluded. In some animals, a midline incision of the brain stem to a depth of about 2.5 mm was made, cutting the direct commissural fibers between the vestibular nuclei. Most recorded neurons were located in the rostral lateral MVN, which previous studies have shown contains some type I neurons which are ocular premotor neurons [Curthoys, unpublished observation].

Results

In the MVN ipsilateral to the ULD (ipsi MVN) the few type I neurons which could be recorded at 0–8 h PO had an average RA of only 2.0 spikes/s.

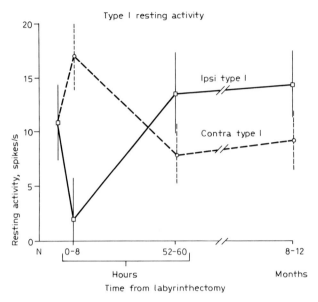

Fig. 1. Type I resting activity in the normal animal (n = 87 neurons) and in animals at different stages following ULD. Solid line represents type I neurons in the MVN ipsilateral to the ULD (ipsi MVN) at 0–8 h (n = 16 neurons), 52–60 h (n = 56) and 8–12 months (n = 114) PO. Dashed line represents type I neurons in the MVN contralateral to the ULD (contra MVN) at the same recording times (n = 126 , 51, 78, respectively). Vertical lines represent two-tailed 95% confidence intervals. N = Normal.

By only 52–60 h PO, type I neurons were encountered more frequently and their average RA was not significantly different from normal; however, it must be emphasized that the frequency of occurrence of type I neurons was still less than normal at all times after ULD. In the MVN contralateral to the ULD (contra MVN), average type I RA was higher than normal at 0–8 h PO, but had decreased to normal by 52–60 h PO (fig. 1). Recordings from the Scarpa's ganglion ipsilateral to the ULD between 52–60 h and 8–12 months PO showed that there was little recovery of RA in peripheral neurons. No responses to horizontal rotation were found. Recordings from neurons in the ipsi MVN following a brain stem midline incision indicated that RA increased. These neurons could not be identified as type I neurons, since no responses to horizontal rotation were found in the ipsi MVN following the midline incision. We presumed that some of these spontaneously active but unresponsive neurons had been type I neurons prior to the midline incision.

Discussion

The recordings made from the Scarpa's ganglion ipsilateral to the ULD in the present experiment show that the recovery of type I RA in the ipsi MVN is not due to a recovery of RA in peripheral neurons and so imply that some change in the CNS must account for the recovery of type I RA in the ipsi MVN [3]. It is unlikely that commissural input was responsible for the recovery of type I RA in the ipsi MVN observed in the present experiment, since the transcerebellar commissures had been removed by midline cerebellar aspiration and a brain stem midline incision produced an increase in the RA of neurons in the ipsi MVN [2]. This finding is consistent with the observation that static symptoms of ULD still compensate following disruption of the brain stem vestibular commissures [4].

What is the origin of the renewed RA of type I neurons in the ipsi MVN? Given the rapid time course of the recovery of RA, axonal sprouting seems an unlikely explanation. Since a similar rapid recovery of RA occurs in other nuclei of the CNS following deafferentation [1], RA may be restored to deafferentated neurons through a functional mechanism, such as increased electrical excitability of the cell membrane [1].

References

1   Calvin, W.H.: Normal repetitive firing and its pathophysiology; in Lockard, Ward, Epilepsy — a window to brain mechanisms, pp. 97–120 (Raven Press, New York 1980).

2   Precht, W.; Shimazu, H.; Markham, C.H.: A mechanism of central compensation of vestibular function following hemilabyrinthectomy. J. Neurophysiol. *29:* 996–1010 (1966).

3   Smith, P.F.; Curthoys, I.S.: Neuronal activity in the ipsilateral medial vestibular nucleus of the guinea pig following unilateral labyrinthectomy. Brain Res. *444:* 308–319 (1988).

4   Smith, P.F.; Darlington, C.L.; Curthoys, I.S.: Vestibular compensation without brainstem commissures in the guinea pig. Neurosci. Lett. *65:* 209–213 (1986).

Dr. I.S. Curthoys, Department of Psychology, University of Sydney, Sydney, NSW 2006 (Australia)

Adv. Oto-Rhino-Laryng., vol. 42, pp. 180–184 (Karger, Basel 1988)

Horizontal Vestibulo-Ocular Reflexes in Humans with Only One Horizontal Semicircular Canal[1]

Philip D. Cremer[a2], *Christopher J. Henderson*[a], *Ian S. Curthoys*[b], *Gabor M. Halmagyi*[a]

[a] Eye and Ear Unit, Department of Neurology, Royal Prince Alfred Hospital, Camperdown; [b] Vestibular Research Laboratory, Department of Psychology, University of Sydney, Sydney, NSW, Australia

How good is the vestibulo-ocular reflex when it is generated by a single semicircular canal? This question goes back to the time of Ewald, who found that ampullopetal endolymph flow caused more vigorous nystagmus than ampullofugal flow in the pigeon's fenestrated horizontal semicircular canal (Ewald's second law). Dohlmann [1] later argued against the validity of Ewald's second law because he could find no asymmetry of rotational nystagmus in unilateral vestibular neurectomy or labyrinthectomy patients. Baloh et al. [2], using head accelerations up to 142 °/s² did, however, find a slight but significant reduction in the gain of the ampullofugal horizontal vestibulo-ocular reflex (AF-HVOR) and predicted that this asymmetry would become more apparent with increasing head accelerations. In this study we have followed their suggestion and, using head accelerations up to 3,000 °/s², have shown a severe, permanent deficit in the AF-HVOR and a slight, sometimes transient, deficit in the ampullopetal horizontal vestibulo-ocular reflex (AP-HVOR) after unilateral vestibular neurectomy. We speculate that it may be possible to explain all these findings on the basis of normal first order vestibular afferent activity.

[1] This work was supported by the National Health and Medical Research Council.
[2] Our thanks to Michael Todd who helped with the equipment and to Cynthia Darlington who helped with the illustrations.

Materials and Method

Horizontal displacement of the head and left eye was recorded in 26 patients using magnetic search coils (Skalar, Delft), during unpredictable, rapid, passive, unidirectional head impulses; before, and from 1 week to 1 year after, therapeutic unilateral vestibular neurectomy for Ménière's disease or intractable vertigo. Each patient sat within an 8-m^3 magnetic field (CNC Engineering, Seattle) fixating a solitary light emitting diode in an otherwise totally darkened room. Without warning the light would be extinguished for about 3 s. This would be the cue for one of the investigators, standing behind the patient, to quickly turn the patient's head about 20° to the right or left. The patient's instructions were to keep fixating the remembered position of the light and to refixate it as soon as it was reilluminated. The peak velocity of head movements varied from 100 to 300 °/s; peak acceleration from 1,000 to 3,000 °/s^2. Head and gaze velocity and acceleration were derived by analog differentiation of the position signals. Eye position was derived by subtracting head from gaze position; this was then differentiated to give eye velocity and acceleration. All signals were displayed on-line on an ink-jet recorder, stored on FM-tape and analyzed off-line using a PDP 11/73 microcomputer.

Results

We found severe permanent deficits in the AF-HVOR of all unilateral vestibular neurectomy patients. Figure 1 shows typical results from a 52-year-old male, 6 weeks after right vestibular neurectomy. In response to a 120 °/s peak velocity rightward head impulse, peak AF-HVOR velocity reaches only about 40 °/s. Furthermore, the eye velocity appears to be a ramp with a constant acceleration of about 300 °/s^2 and a delay of peak eye velocity relative to peak head velocity of about 80 ms. Figure 1 also shows a slight deficit of the AP-HVOR: peak eye velocity is only about 90 °/s compared to a peak head velocity of about 115 °/s and peak eye acceleration is about 300 °/s^2 less than peak head acceleration but unlike with the AF-HVOR there is no delay. These two HVOR patterns to an impulsive head stimulus could be found, basically unaltered, up to 12 months after unilateral vestibular neurectomy.

Discussion

Our findings confirm previous observations of a permanent deficit in the AF-HVOR following unilateral vestibular neurectomy and show that it is more severe than previously thought [2]. Figure 2 compares an impulsive stimulus of the type used in this study with a standard vestibular stimulus (in

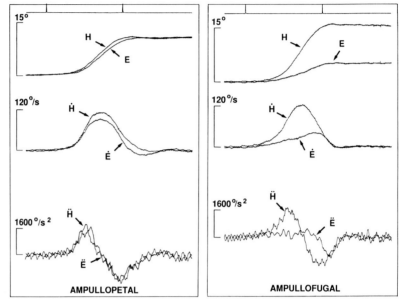

Fig. 1. Ampullofugal (on left) and ampullopetal (on right) horizontal VOR during 1,600 °/s² peak acceleration head impulses, 6 weeks after unilateral vestibular neurectomy. There is a severe deficit of the ampullofugal VOR with saturation of the eye acceleration and a delay in its zero crossing relative to head acceleration. There is also a mild deficit in the peak velocity and acceleration of the ampullopetal VOR.

this case a 0.2-Hz sinusoid with 200 °/s² peak-to-peak acceleration) of the type used in previous studies which have failed to show a deficit of the AF-HVOR. We agree with Baloh et al. [2] that fast head movements are required to show the true performance of the AF-HVOR and that previous studies have used stimuli that were too slow compared with the speed of natural head movements.

If silencing of first order vestibular afferents by large head accelerations, as described by Goldberg and Fernandez [3] in the squirrel monkey, does indeed, as suggested by Baloh et al., [2], explain the AF-HVOR deficit in humans after unilateral vestibular neurectomy, it is surprising to find that it is eye acceleration rather than eye velocity that appears to saturate. The firing rate of most regularly discharging first order vestibular afferents is a function of head, and therefore by implication of eye velocity [4]. It would, therefore, be reasonable to expect that silencing of first order afferents would lead to a saturation of AF-HVOR velocity rather than of acceleration. The fact that it

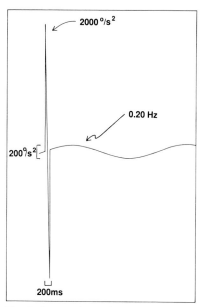

Fig. 2. Comparison of an impulsive stimulus (as used in this study) which has a period of 200 ms and a peak-to-peak magnitude of 4,000 °/s² with a typical vestibular stimulus which has a period of 5 s and peak-to-peak magnitude of 200 °/s².

is eye acceleration rather than velocity which appears to saturate, raises the possibility that the AF-HVOR is dominated by the firing of first order afferents which signal head acceleration (i.e. cupular velocity), rather than head velocity (i.e. cupular displacement). The explanation of the mild AP-HVOR deficit is equally speculative, but could involve loss of normal commissural disinhibition by lesioned side type I vestibular nucleus neurons, of type I vestibular neurons on the intact side [5].

References

1   Dohlmann, G.F.: On the case for repeal of Ewald's second law. Acta oto-lar., suppl. 159, pp. 15–24 (1960).
2   Baloh, R.W.; Honrubia, V.; Konrad, H.R.: Ewald's second law re-evaluated. Acta oto-lar. *83:* 475–479 (1977).
3   Goldberg, J.M.; Fernandez, C.: Physiology of peripheral neurons innervating semi-circular canals of the squirrel monkey. I. Resting discharge and response to constant accelerations. J. Neurophysiol. *34:* 635–659 (1971).

4   Fernandez, C.; Goldberg, J.: Physiology of peripheral neurons innervating semi-
    circular canals of squirrel monkey. II. Response to sinusoidal stimulation and
    dynamics of the peripheral vestibular system. J. Neurophysiol. *34:* 661–675 (1971).
5   Markham, C.H.; Yagi, T.; Curthoys, I.S.: The contribution of the contralateral
    labyrinth to second order vestibular neuronal activity in the cat. Brain Res. *138:* 99–
    109 (1977).

Dr. G.M. Halmagyi, Eye and Ear Unit, Department of Neurology,
RPA Hospital, Camperdown, Sydney NSW 2050 (Australia)

Adv. Oto-Rhino-Laryng., vol. 42, pp. 185–189 (Karger, Basel 1988)

The Role of Cervical Inputs in Compensation of Unilateral Labyrinthectomized Patients

Yuzuru Kobayashi, Toshiaki Yagi, Tomokazu Kamio

Department of Otolaryngology, Nippon Medical School, Bunkyo-ku, Tokyo, Japan

Introduction

It has been known that the proprioceptors of muscles and joints of the neck play an important role in the control of eye movements as well as in the postural adjustment. Nystagmus was demonstrated after dissection of the dorsal root of the cervical spine in cats and rabbits [1–3]. In human subjects, eye deviation and nystagmus were also provoked by neck torsion [4–9]. These eye movements induced by stimulation of cervical sensory organs are called cervico-ocular reflex.

In human subjects, we previously demonstrated clear nystagmus by vibratory stimulation of the dorsal neck [10]. The frequency and slow phase eye velocity of the neck vibration nystagmus in patients with unilateral labyrinthine dysfunction are greater than those in normal subjects. The neck vibration also modulates the caloric nystagmus in patients with unilateral labyrinthine dysfunction, but has no effect on the caloric nystagmus in normal subjects. These results suggest that the cervico-vestibular interaction is stronger in patients with unilateral labyrinthine dysfunction than that in normal subjects.

In animal experiments, it has been reported that the sensory inputs from the neck proprioceptors modulate the process of the vestibular compensation after unilateral labyrinthectomy [11, 12]. Thus, in the present study, we investigated the course of spontaneous and neck vibration nystagmus in 2 patients with unilateral labyrinthectomy to clarify the role of cervical inputs in the vestibular compensation.

Method

Two patients who underwent translabyrinthine acoustic neuroma resection were the subjects of this investigation. The caloric test showed hypofunction in both cases before the labyrinthectomy. The spontaneous nystagmus was recorded under eye-open conditions in the dark by electronystagmography (ENG). The neck vibration nystagmus was observed behind Frenzel's glasses while the ENG was recorded simultaneously. The observation period was more than 2 years after the labyrinthectomy. For vibrating the dorsal neck, a specially designed vibrator was used. The stimulation frequency of the vibrator was 125 Hz. Vibratory stimulation was applied to both sides of the neck, the right side during head turning to the left, and the left side during head turning to the right in the supine position. The patients had no disturbance of the central nervous system before or after surgery.

Results

In one patient whose nystagmus was followed up for 27 months after surgery, the average slow phase eye velocity of spontaneous nystagmus before undergoing labyrinthectomy was 7.5 °/s. The velocity of the nystagmus decreased quite rapidly, 6.1 °/s at one month and 3.1 °/s at 3 months after the surgery. It then decreased gradually to 2.5 °/s at 27 months after labyrinthectomy. On the contrary, the slow phase eye velocity of the neck vibration nystagmus increased after the labyrinthectomy. The average slow phase velocity was 2.1 °/s before surgery and increased rapidly, 5.7 °/s at one month and 8.3 °/s at 2 months after surgery; i.e. the slow phase velocity of the neck-induced nystagmus was almost the same as that of spontaneous nystagmus at one month after surgery and greater than that at 2 months after surgery. Although the slow phase eye velocity of neck vibration nystagmus did not vary greatly with a few exceptions thereafter, the velocity was always greater than that of the spontaneous nystagmus (fig. 1).

In the second patient whose nystagmus was followed up for 24 months after labyrinthectomy, the average slow phase eye velocity of spontaneous nystagmus before surgery was 6.6 °/s. The velocity of the nystagmus, however, did not decrease, 10.0 °/s at 9 months and 7.3 °/s at 24 months after surgery. The average slow phase velocity of the neck vibration nystagmus was 2.8 °/s, before surgery. Although the slow phase velocity increased after the labyrinthectomy, it was always smaller than that of spontaneous nystagmus until 9 months after labyrinthectomy. After that the velocity of the neck vibration nystagmus became slightly greater than that of spontaneous nystagmus (fig. 2).

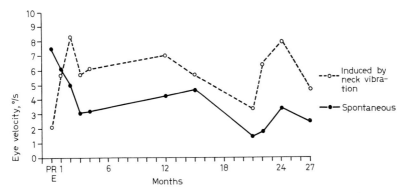

Fig. 1. Eye velocity of nystagmus before and after labyrinthectomy (case 1).

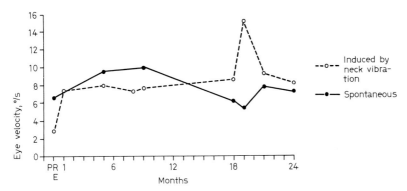

Fig. 2. Eye velocity of nystagmus before and after labyrinthectomy (case 2).

Discussion

Previously, we reported that the inputs from neck proprioceptors play an important role in the control of eye movements in patients with unilateral labyrinthine dysfunction [10]. Even in the compensated stage following unilateral labyrinthine dysfunction, the sensory input modulation from the neck proprioceptors by the neck vibration induced marked nystagmus; in other words, the neck vibration caused the discompensation [10]. In the present study, the slow phase eye velocity of the neck vibration nystagmus increased after labyrinthectomy in both cases. This result suggests that the cervical sensory inputs become more prominent for controlling the eye movements at the compensation stage after the hemilabyrinthectomy. There was, however, a difference in the course of slow phase eye velocity of the neck vibration nystagmus between these 2 cases. In the first case, the slow phase eye velocity of the spontaneous nystagmus decreased after labyrinthectomy and that of neck vibration nystagmus increased markedly. On the other hand, in the second case, the slow phase eye velocity of the spontaneous nystagmus did not decrease after labyrinthectomy and that of neck vibration nystagmus increased slightly. The decrease in the slow phase velocity of the spontaneous nystagmus is probably due to the development of the compensation process in the vestibulo-ocular pathways, so that the level of the vestibular compensation in the first case is better than that in the second case. Modulation of the sensory inputs from the neck proprioceptors by neck vibration induced marked nystagmus in the first patient who should have gained better vestibular compensation than the second patient after the hemilabyrinthectomy. Thus, it can be speculated that the cervical sensory inputs play an important role in the process of vestibular compensation.

References

1 Biemond, A.: On a new form of experimental positional-nystagmus in the rabbit and its clinical value. Proc. Akad. Wet. 42: 370–375 (1939).
2 Biemond, A.: Further observation about the cervical form of positional-nystagmus and its anatomical base. Proc. Akad. Wet. 43: 901–906 (1940).
3 Biemond, A.; De Jong, J.M.B.V.: On cervical nystagmus and related disorders. Brain 92: 437–458 (1969).
4 Bárány, R.: Augenbewegungen durch Thoraxbewegungen ausgelöst. Zentbl. Physiol. 20: 298–303 (1906).
5 Bos, J.H.; Philipszoon, A.J.: Neck torsion nystagmus. Practica oto-rhino-lar. 25:177–187 (1936).
6 Philipszoon, A.J.: Compensatory eye movements and eye nystagmus provoked by stimulation of the vestibular organs and the cervical nerve roots. Practica oto-rhino-lar. 24: 193–202 (1962).
7 Bos, J.H.: On vestibular nystagmus without causative endolymphatic displacement; academic thesis, Amsterdam (1962).
8 Jongkees, L.B.W.: Cervical vertigo. Laryngoscope 79: 1473–1484 (1969).
9 Suzuki, J.; Takemori, S.: Eye movement induced from the spinal nerve. Equil. Res., suppl. 2, pp. 33–40 (1970).
10 Kobayashi, Y.; Yagi, T.; Kamio, T.: Cervico-vestibular interaction in eye movements. Auris, Nasus, Larynx, Tokyo 13: 87–95 (1986).
11 Schaefer, K.P.; Meyer, D.L.; Wilhelms, G.: Somatosensory and cerebellar influences on compensation of labyrinthine lesions; in Pompeiano, Reflex control of posture

and movement, pp. 591–598 (Elsevier, North-Holland Biomedical Press, Amsterdam 1979).
12 Pettorossi Vioto, E.; Petrosini, L.: Tonic cervical influences on eye nystagmus following hemilabyrinthectomy. Brain Res. *324:* 11–19 (1984).

Yuzuru Kobayashi, MD, Department of Otolaryngology, Nippon Medical School, 1-1-5 Sendagi, Bunkyo-ku, Tokyo 113 (Japan)

Adv. Oto-Rhino-Laryng., vol. 42, pp. 190–194 (Karger, Basel 1988)

Primary Position Upbeat Nystagmus in Man and Cats

Koji Harada[a], *Isao Kato*[b], *Yoshio Koike*[a], *Yo Kimura*[a],
Tadashi Nakamura[a], *Jin Watanabe*[a]

[a]Department of Otolaryngology, Yamagata University School of Medicine,
Yamagata; [b]Department of Otolaryngology, St. Marianna University School of
Medicine, Kawasaki, Japan

Introduction

It is said that primary position upbeat nystagmus (PPUN) has been associated with lesions of the midbrain, cerebellar vermis, brachium conjunctivum or lower brain stem on clinical grounds. In previous reports, however, the precise localization remains unclear. The purpose of this study is to clarify the localizing value of the PPUN by use of clinical findings in a patient and experimental lesions in cats.

Case Report

A 39-year-old woman was admitted on the seventh day after a sudden onset of dysarthria and vertical oscillopsia. The patient had tongue deviation to the right and slight atrophy on the right side of the tongue with simultaneous palatal weakness. Eye movements were full, but there was prominent upbeat nystagmus that persisted in all directions of gaze. Upbeat nystagmus in the primary position has an amplitude of 5–8° and a frequency of 2 Hz. While in upward gaze, the amplitude of the nystagmus increased to 10°, and frequency to 3 Hz. In downward gaze, the amplitude of the nystagmus decreased to 3–5° and frequency to 1 Hz (fig. 1). No other abnormal signs were observed neurologically.

The EOG test was performed for the measurement of the eye movements on both horizontal and vertical axes. Vertical pursuit eye movements indicated saccadic upward pursuit and normal downward tracking. The patient followed the upward optokinetic stimuli, but showed extreme velocity limitation, while downward optokinetic stimuli produced normal up-OKN. Horizontal eye movements (pursuit and OKN) were quantitatively normal.

Vertebral angiography and computed tomography did not indicate abnormalities. The CSF only was slightly xanthochromic. Her condition improved rapidly. The PPUN

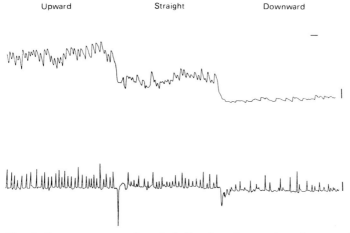

Fig. 1. Gaze nystagmus of vertical directions in a patient. In upward gaze, the nystagmus increases, and in downward gaze, decreases. The upper trace is a DC-EOG recording; the lower trace, eye velocity (time constant 0.03).

disappeared on the seventh hospital day. The tongue deviation completely recovered, but slight atrophy and palatal weakness remained. At that time, all eye movements of both horizontal and vertical axes were normal.

Neurological findings and laboratory examinations suggest that the patient had a discrete vascular lesion in the lower dorsal brain stem involving the hypoglossal nucleus and adjacent structures, and that PPUN may result from a lesion of this region.

Materials and Methods in Experimental Research

In 10 cats, the EOG test was performed before the floor of the fourth ventricle was destroyed electrolytically in order to produce PPUN. The occipital bone was removed, and then the cerebellar vermis was carefully elevated by spatula to expose the floor of the caudal fourth ventricle. Unilateral lesions were produced in 5 cats. The remaining 5 cats had bilateral lesions. After follow-up studies of eye movements recorded with DC-EOG were completed, the extent of the lesions was determined by serial frozen sections at 600-µm intervals.

Results

In 5 cats who had unilateral lesions of the floor of the fourth ventricle, PPUN was never seen. Two of the remaining 5 cats, who had bilateral lesions, showed PPUN. In 2 cats (110, 126) with PPUN, the oculomotor behavior was similar in spite of differences in the extent of lesions. Upbeat nystagmus in a primary position in light consisted of an amplitude of 8–13° and a frequency of 2 Hz. In total darkness, the amplitude of the upbeat nystagmus increased to 12–15°, and the frequency unchanged. Change of the head positions affected both amplitude and frequency of the upbeat nystagmus. In vertical optokinetic nystagmus (OKN), during upward OK stimuli, down-OKN was not generated and spontaneous upbeat nystagmus was seen. On the other hand, up-OKN increased to be enhanced by spontaneous nystagmus. In vertical vestibulo-ocular reflex (VOR), the gain of the upward VOR decreased remarkably and downward VOR increased by the upbeat nystagmus. Horizontal OKN and VOR remained normal. These lesions selectively impaired vertical eye movements and did not affect horizontal eye movements.

In cat 110 with PPUN, the fourth ventricle lesions were larger than those in cat 126. There was symmetrical destruction of the midline structures, deep to the fourth ventricle and involving the prepositus hypoglossal nucleus (PH), Roller's nucleus (RN), the intercalatus nucleus (IC), the medial longitudinal fasciculus (MLF), the dorsal tegmentum (DT) and the hypoglossal nucleus (XII) symmetrically on both sides. The abducens nucleus and the vestibular nuclei (VN) were spared.

On the other hand, in cat 126, the extent of the lesions wasa smaller than those in cat 110. The PH was damaged on both sides, but the MLF was impaired unilaterally. Roller's nucleus, the IC, the vagal nucleus and the hypoglossal nucleus were spared. Histological findings in 3 typical cats without PPUN are shown in table I. Unilateral PH lesions (cat 119) and bilateral MLF lesions (cat 122 and 123) did not develop PPUN (table I).

Discussion

It is said that both upbeat and downbeat nystagmus may result from a defect in the vertical smooth pursuit system [1, 2]. In our case, upward pursuit was totally damaged and downward pursuit was normal. The subsequent report, however, criticized this theory, and that pursuit asymmetry was interpreted as the result rather than the cause [3].

In this experiment, the produced PPUN in cats was affected by the vestibular input (change of the head positions) and the condition in light. From this finding, PPUN will be one of the 'central vestibular nystagmus'.

Table I. Nuclei and fiber tracts lesioned in cats

Lesion site	With PPUN		Without PPUN		
	110	126	122	123	119
PH	B	B	U	—	U
IC	B	—	U	—	U
RN	B	—	U	—	U
XN	B	—	U	—	U
XII N	B	—	U	—	U
MLF	B	U	B	B	U
DT	B	U	U	U	U
VN	—	—	—	—	U

B = Bilateral lesions; U = unilateral lesions; — = no lesion; PH = prepositus hypoglossal nucleus; IC = intercalatus nucleus; RN = Roller's nucleus; XN = vagal nucleus; XII N = hypoglossal nucleus; MLF = medial longitudinal fasciculus; DT = dorsal tegmentum; VN = vestibular nuclei.

Therefore, vertical pursuit asymmetry may be interpreted as the result of PPUN.

From the histological analysis in the lesions at the level of the caudal fourth ventricle, in order that PPUN may be developed, it will be necessary that the PH is destroyed bilaterally.

Morphologic [4] and physiologic [5] studies reveal reciprocal anatomic connections of the PH with nearly all known brain stem nuclei and cerebellum responsible for oculomotor function. Neurons in the PH receive vestibular input directly and this excites monosynaptically oculomotor neurons, especially in relation to vertical eye movements [5]. In the observations, we suggest that the PH lesion could result in a tonic imbalance for eye positions and eye movements of the vertical axis, resulting in an upbeat nystagmus in man and cats.

References

1   Gilman, N.; Baloh, R.W.; Tomiyasu, U.: Primary position upbeat nystagmus. Neurology *27*: 294–298 (1977).
2   Zee, D.; Friendlich, A.; Robinson, D.: The mechanism of downbeat nystagmus. Archs Neurol. *30*: 227–237 (1974).

3   Baloh, R.W.; Spooner, J.W.: Downbeat nystagmus: a type of central vestibular nystagmus. Neurology *31:* 304–310 (1981).
4   Brodal, A.: The perihypoglossal nuclei in the macaque monkey and the chimpanzee. J. comp. Neurol. *218:* 257–269 (1983).
5   Baker, R.: The nucleus prepositus hypoglossi; in Brooks, Bajandas, Eye movements, pp. 145–178 (Plenum Publishing, New York 1976).

Koji Harada, MD, Department of Otolaryngology, Yamagata University
School of Medicine, Yamagata 990-23 (Japan)

Adv. Oto-Rhino-Laryng., vol. 42, pp. 195–201 (Karger, Basel 1988)

Neurotological Differentiation between Cerebellar and Brain Stem Lesions

H. Mineda, H. Ishizaki, K. Umemura, M. Nozue

Department of Otorhinolaryngology, School of Medicine, Hamamatsu University, Shizuoka, Japan

Introduction

Although the diagnosis of intracranial diseases has considerably advanced, the differential diagnosis between cerebellar and brain stem lesions remains quite difficult in many cases. However, the recent advances in neurotology seem to give us some useful information. We then comparatively analyzed the neurotological findings associated with cerebellar and brain stem lesions.

Materials and Methods

We analyzed 41 cases. Twenty-six cerebellar lesions included 3 cerebellitis, 6 tumors, 13 hemorrhages and 4 infarcts, and 14 brain stem lesions included 5 tumors, 4 hemorrhages and 6 infarcts.

And we analyzed such eye movements as saccades, smooth pursuits and optokinetic nystagmus. The saccade was analyzed not only qualitatively but also quantitatively. The velocity of the saccade was also measured. Horizontal eye movements were recorded bitemporally. Each had a full range of extraocular movement at the time of recordings. After calibration, the following eye movements were recorded. To read saccades, the target 30° was lighted alternately. To record smooth pursuits, the light was moved with a sinusoid pattern 30° apart. To test optokinetic nystagmus, an Ohm-type drum was rotated, from 0 to approximately 180 °/s and then to 0 °/s with an acceleration and deceleration of ± 4 °/s^2. The velocity of the induced optokinetic nystagmus was recorded with a slow chart speed of 1 mm/s, namely the optokinetic pattern (OKP) test.

Furthermore, recovery processes of eye movements in patients with cerebellar or brain stem lesions typically were demonstrated.

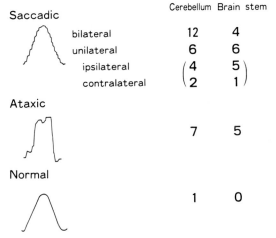

Fig. 1. Types of smooth pursuit.

Table I. Findings of saccade in 26 patients

	Cerebellum	Brain stem
Dysmetria		
+	24	4
–	2	11
Maximum velocity		
Decreased	5	12
Bilateral	2	9
Unilateral	3	3
Ipsilateral	2	3
Contralateral	1	0
Normal	21	3

Results

Smooth Pursuit

To qualitatively analyze smooth pursuits, we divided them into 3 patterns: namely saccadic, ataxic and normal. The saccadic pattern was divided into bilateral or unilateral and the latter was further divided into 2 groups, depending on the direction, one toward the side of lesion (ipsilateral) and the other toward the intact side (contralateral).

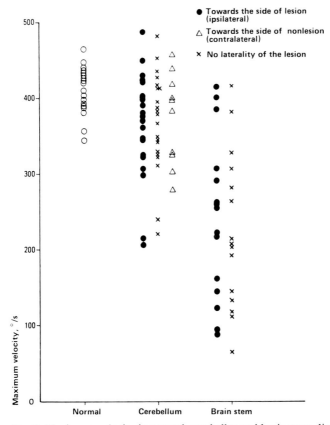

Fig. 2. Maximum velocity in normal, cerebellar and brain stem disorders.

With cerebellar lesions, 18 cases showed saccadic patterns among which 12 were bilateral and 6 were unilateral, and 7 others showed ataxic patterns.

With brain stem lesions, 10 cases showed saccadic and 5 showed ataxic patterns. As for the direction, ipsilateral was commoner than contralateral with both lesions (fig. 1).

Saccade

Twenty-four of 26 cases with cerebellar lesions showed dysmetric eye movements, while 11 of 15 cases with brain stem lesions did not. As for the maximum velocity, with cerebellar lesions, 21 cases showed normal, while 5 showed decreased velocities: 2 in both directions and 3 in a unilateral

	Cerebellum	Brain stem
Suppressed	17	13
lesion side = nonlesion side	5	9
>	8	3
<	4	1
Normal	9	2

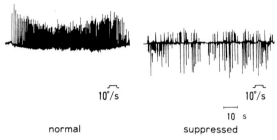

10°/s   10°/s

                               10 s

normal   suppressed

Fig. 3. Findings of the OKP test.

direction. With brain stem lesions, 12 cases showed decreased velocities: 9 in both and 3 in ipsilateral directions (table I).

The mean maximum velocity in 9 normal subjects was 410.9 °/s. The maximum velocity with cerebellar lesions did not differ significantly from that of normal subjects, but was slower with brain stem lesions (fig. 2).

Optokinetic Nystagmus — OKP Test

With cerebellar lesions, the optokinetic nystagmus was suppressed in 17 cases but was normal in 9. With brain stem lesions, it was suppressed in 13 cases, but was normal in 2. As for the directional preponderance, in 8 cases with cerebellar lesions the optokinetic nystagmus was more suppressed to the side of the lesion. On the other hand, 9 cases with brain stem lesions did not show the directional preponderance (fig. 3).

Recovery Processes

The recovery process of eye movements (smooth pursuit and saccade) was shown in a patient with a left cerebellar hemisphere hemorrhage. After one day, the smooth pursuit was bilaterally saccadic and the saccade was followed by dysmetric eye movements of overshoot. After 2 weeks, mild saccadic movements were present during the smooth pursuit and a few overshoots were present during the saccade. After one month, the smooth

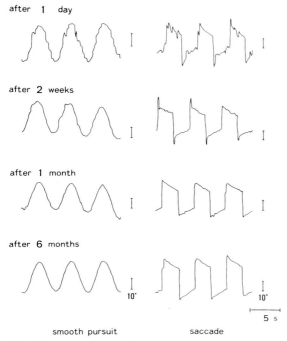

after 1   day

after 2 weeks

after 1 month

after 6 months

10°   10°

5 s

smooth pursuit   saccade

Fig. 4. Recovery process of eye movements (smooth pursuit and saccade) in a patient with a cerebellar hemorrhage.

pursuit was almost normal and the saccade had only residual overshoots (fig. 4). In a patient with a pontine hemorrhage, the smooth pursuit was ataxic and the saccade was slower to the left side after 6 months. After 2 years, although the nystagmus was superimposed, the smooth pursuit showed some recovery and the saccade became somewhat faster (fig. 5).

The recovery processes of optokinetic nystagmus in patients with the cerebellar or the pontine hemorrhages were shown. With the pontine lesion, the optokinetic nystagmus was markedly suppressed throughout the course. With the cerebellar lesion, although the optokinetic nystagmus was suppressed after one day, it recovered well and became normal after 4 weeks (fig. 6).

Discussion

In this report, we analyzed saccades, smooth pursuits and optokinetic nystagmus to observe the neurotological differentiation between cerebellar and brain stem lesions, and discussed their recovery processes.

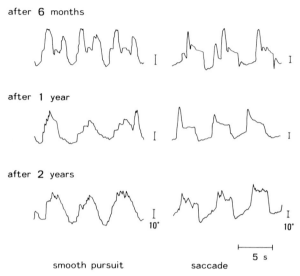

Fig. 5. Recovery process of eye movements (smooth pursuit and saccade) in a patient with a pontine hemorrhage.

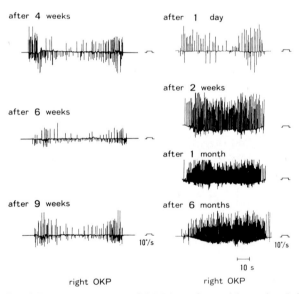

Fig. 6. Recovery processes of OKP in patients with pontine (left) or cerebellar (right) hemorrhages.

During the smooth pursuit, the abnormality was found in 96.2% (25 of 26 cases) with cerebellar lesions and in 100% (15 of 15 cases) with brain stem lesions. It is suggested that the cerebellum and the brain stem networks are involved in the mechanisms of the smooth pursuit movement [1, 2]; however, qualitative analysis does not reveal characteristic differences between them. During the saccade we examined the dysmetria and the maximum velocity. The velocity was normal but was followed by dysmetric eye movements with cerebellar lesions, while with brain stem lesions the saccade was slower but was not followed by dysmetric eye movements. Therefore, it might be thought that cerebellar lesions primarily affect saccade accuracy; on the other hand, brain stem lesions result in slowing velocity [2–4].

During the optokinetic nystagmus it seemed to be suppressed by both lesions. But brain stem lesions tended to be markedly suppressed, and cerebellar lesions showed early recovery despite the abnormalities of saccade and smooth pursuit.

Clinically, cerebellar lesions may not be considered to cause the suppression of optokinetic nystagmus, without the compression of the brain stem.

With both lesions the abnormalities of smooth pursuit, saccade and optokinetic nystagmus were more markedly observed ipsilaterally than contralaterally [5]. In recovery processes, cerebellar lesions showed earlier recovery than brain stem lesions. It might be thought that the brain stem affected eye movements more strongly. From these results, neurotological examinations seem to be useful in evaluating the localizations of lesions and their recovery processes.

References

1   Nemet, P.; Ron, S.: Cerebellar role in smooth pursuit movement. Documenta ophth. *43:* 101–107 (1977).
2   Baloh, R.W.; Honrubia, V.; Sills, A.: Eye-tracking and optokinetic nystagmus. Ann. Otol. *86:* 108–114 (1977).
3   Wennmo, C.; Pyykkö, I.: Velocity patterns of eye movements in brainstem lesions. Differential diagnosis of vertigo, pp. 219–233 (de Gruyter, Berlin 1980).
4   Baloh, R.W.; Konrad, H.R.; Sills, A.W.; Honrubia, V.: The saccade velocity test. Neurology *25:* 1071–1076 (1975).
5   Ron, S.; Nemet, P.: The cerebellum involvement in the generation of saccades. Documenta ophth. *43:* 109–114 (1977).

H. Mineda, MD, Department of Otorhinolaryngology, Hamamatsu University School of Medicine, 3600 Handa-cho, Hamamatsu 431-31 (Japan)

Adv. Oto-Rhino-Laryng., vol. 42, pp. 202–204 (Karger, Basel 1988)

Diagnostic Confirmation of Lesions in Cerebellar Peduncles by Combined Use of Optokinetic Nystagmus and Fixation-Suppression of Caloric Nystagmus

I. Kato[a], *J. Watanabe*[b], *T. Nakamura*[b], *K. Harada*[b], *Y. Hasegawa*[b], *R. Kanayama*[b]

[a]Department of Otolaryngology, St. Marianna University School of Medicine, Sugao, Kawasaki; [b]Department of Otolaryngology, Yamagata University School of Medicine, Yamagata, Japan

The neurophysiological studies of the cerebellum have disclosed that some floccular Purkinje cells increase their firing rates responding to high velocity optokinetic nystagmus (OKN) stimulation above 60 °/s with slow phase ipsilateral to the recording side, and similar increases in firing rates are recognized with suppression of contralateral slow phase of vestibular nystagmus during visual-vestibular interaction [3]. In accordance with this fact, lesions of the flocculus result in limitation of slow phase OKN at higher stimulus velocity toward the lesion side in cats [2] and reduce the ability of monkeys to cancel vestibular nystagmus with slow phase toward the side contralateral to the lesion during visual-vestibular interaction [4].

Based on these single cell and lesion studies, 17 patients with unilateral cerebellar lesions were investigated. None of the signs concerning floccular lesions observed in animal experiments were demonstrated from the EOG findings, showing bilateral OKN velocity limitation from lower stimulus ranges, failure of fixation-suppression on both sides and saccadic pursuit on both sides [1].

In the present experiment EOG assessment was made in patients with lesions of cerebellar peduncles in search for the possibility of neurophysiological evidence of the cerebellum, demonstrated in animal experiments.

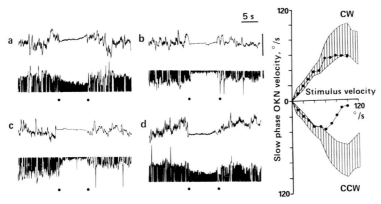

Fig. 1. Caloric nystagmus (left) and gain of slow phase OKN velocity (right). The upper traces in *a–d* are DC-EOG recordings; the second traces in each series, slow phase velocity. Upward trace deflections represent eye movement to the right. The EOG in *a* and *b* are caloric nystagmus induced by right ear stimulation with cold (*a*) and hot water (*b*), and those in *c* and *d*, by left ear stimulation. Black dots in each trace indicate a period during ocular fixation. Calibrations shown farthest to the right in *b* are 20° for the EOG and 20 °/s for the velocity trace. Fixation-suppression of caloric nystagmus with rightward slow phase is lost (*a, d*). On the right, the hatched area indicates mean ± SD based on 17 normal persons. Leftward slow phase OKN velocity is saturated at a stimulus velocity greater than 40 °/s.

Materials and Methods

Of 2,240 patients, 28 were diagnosed as having discrete unilateral lesions in the brain stem by both neurological signs and symptoms and CT. In 7 of 28 patients, lesions in the cerebellar peduncles were confirmed by identifying lesions through CT and having cerebellar signs on the same side. Horizontal eye movements were recorded with DC-EOG. Both slow phase OKN and fixation-suppression of caloric nystagmus were evaluated using slow phase velocity according to our criteria [1].

Results

Slow phase OKN velocity was limited toward the lesion side, whereas fixation-suppression of caloric nystagmus with slow phase velocity was lost toward the side contraleral to the lesion in all 7 patients who had lesions either in the superior or the middle cerebellar peduncle (fig. 1).

Discussion

In the previous paper, well-defined cerebellar lesions on one side were large enough to occupy the cerebellar hemisphere. In such patients, EOG abnormalities characteristic of cerebellectomized animals [2–4] were rarely detected, suggesting large mass effects upon the brain stem on both sides from the points of EOG abnormalities [1].

Consequently, it can be emphasized that EOG abnormalities, as shown in figure 1, are solely ascribed to lesions of either the superior or the middle cerebellar peduncle.

The present EOG findings — that the direction of OKN limitation and failure of fixation-suppression is dissociate in patients with lesions of cerebellar peduncles — are interpreted as an abnormality of neural events of the cerebellum demonstrated in animal experiments. Therefore, the combined use of OKN and fixation-suppression of caloric nystagmus provides a valuable diagnostic information on lesions of cerebellar peduncles.

References

1   Kato, I.; Watanabe, J.; Nakamura, T.; et al.: Electronystagmographic assessment of cerebellar lesions. Auris, Nasus, Larynx, Tokyo *13:* suppl., II, pp. S171–S180 (1986).
2   Precht, W.; Strata, P.: On the pathway mediating optokinetic responses in vestibular nucleus neurons. Neuroscience *5:* 777–787 (1980).
3   Waespe,f W.; Henn, V.: Visual-vestibular interaction in the flocculus of the alert monkey. II. Purkinje cell activity. Exp. Brain Res. *43:* 349–360 (1981).
4   Zee, D.S.; Yamazaki, A.; Butler, P.H.; Gücer, G.: Effect of ablation of flocculus and paraflocculus on eye movements in primates. J. Neurophysiol. *46:* 878–899 (1981).

I. Kato, MD, Department of Otolaryngology, St. Marianna University
School of Medicine, 213 Sugao, Kawasaki (Japan)

Adv. Oto-Rhino-Laryng., vol. 42, pp. 205–209 (Karger, Basel 1988)

Studies on Voluntary and Reflexive Optokinetic Nystagmus in Cerebellar Disorders: With Qualitative and Quantitative Tests

Keisuke Mizuta, Takashi Tokita, Hideo Miyata, Masami Yanagida, Kazuhiko Amano

Department of Otorhinolaryngology, Gifu University School of Medicine, Gifu, Japan

This report describes the characteristics of optokinetic nystagmus (OKN) in patients with cerebellar disorders.

Methods and Materials

An Ohm-type rotating cylinder was used to examine the horizontal OKN. The cylinder measured 2 m in diameter and 2 m in height. Twelve vertical stripes were drawn at equal intervals on its inner surface. The cylinder was rotated with an electric motor at an angular acceleration of $2°/s^2$ for 90 s.

OKN was examined using two methods. (1) The examinees were instructed to look at the stripes so as to count them, one by one. The OKN induced by this method was Schau-nystagmus, as described by Ter Braak [1936]. We termed this voluntary OKN. (2) The examinees were instructed to stare vacantly ahead. The OKN induced by this method was Stier-nystagmus, which we termed reflexive OKN.

OKN was recorded by electronystagmography and analyzed with a PDP-11 computer both qualitatively and quantitatively. Qualitatively, nystagmus waves and stripe movements were displayed in superimposition on a cathode ray tube. From the relation between the two, the ocular ability to catch and follow the stripes was evaluated [Tokita et al., 1983]. Quantitatively, the number of beats, the average amplitude and the average eye speed of nystagmus for each 10-second period were calculated. The values obtained in each clinical case were compared with the normal range [Tokita et al., 1975].

The subjects studied were as follows. (1) A patient with astrocytoma of the right cerebellar hemisphere. (2) A patient with Arnold-Chiari malformation. This case showed downbeat nystagmus, ocular dysmetria, rebound nystagmus, saccadic pursuit and failure of visual suppression, indicating disturbance of the posterior vermis and the flocculus. (3) A patient with cerebellar atrophy. This case showed downbeat nystagmus in positioning and failure of visual suppression, suggesting dysfunction of the flocculus. (4) A patient

Voluntary OKN

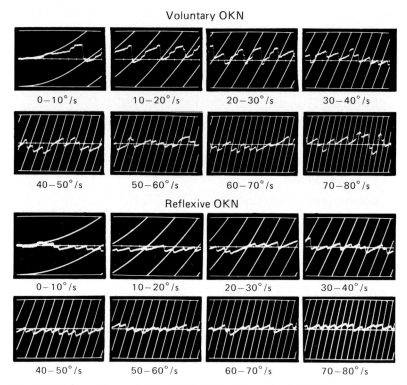

Fig. 1. OKN in a patient with Arnold-Chiari malformation (cylinder rotation to the right).

with olivo-ponto-cerebellar atrophy. This case showed atrophy of the brain stem and cerebellum by computed tomography.

Results

OKN of the Patient with Astrocytoma of the Right Cerebellar Hemisphere. In voluntary and reflexive OKN, no abnormalities were noted either qualitatively or quantitatively.

OKN of the Patient with Arnold-Chiari Malformation. The upper column of figure 1 shows the qualitative analysis of voluntary OKN. Pursuit eye movement was delayed and saccadic movements were noted in stripe pursuit. When the cylinder speed exceeded 20°/s, ocular dysmetria was

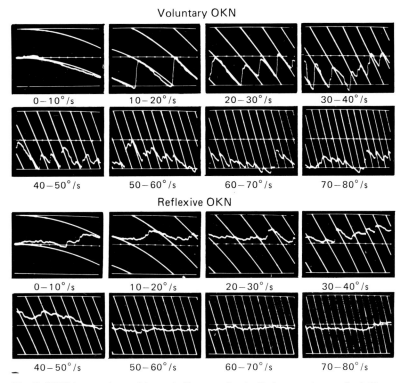

Fig. 2. OKN in a patient with cerebellar atrophy (cylinder rotation to the left).

observed in the eye movement for the target catch. The lower column of figure 1 shows reflexive OKN. Nystagmus did not occur actively, but nystagmus waves were regular. Quantitatively, in reflexive OKN, the number of beats and the eye speed in the slow phase were decreased.

OKN of the Patient with Cerebellar Atrophy. The upper column of figure 2 shows the qualitative analysis of voluntary OKN. Pursuit eye movement corresponded to the target movement at a cylinder speed of up to 30°/s. When the cylinder speed exceeded 30°/s, pursuit eye movement was delayed. However, voluntary OKN did not indicate disorders of wave form, as was noted with the second case. The lower column shows reflexive OKN. The amplitude of nystagmus decreased and nystagmus occurred sporadically. Quantitatively, when the cylinder speed exceeded 60°/s, the number of beats and the eye speed in the slow phase were markedly decreased in voluntary

OKN. In reflexive OKN, the eye speed in the slow phase was decreased at all cylinder speeds.

OKN of the Patient with Olivo-Ponto-Cerebellar Atrophy. Qualitatively, both voluntary and reflexive OKN indicated irregularity of nystagmus waves and did not occur actively.

Discussion

In the present patient suffering from disorder of the cerebellar hemisphere, OKN abnormalities were not noted, as reported by Hishida [1984]. Kase et al. [1980] have reported that the posterior vermis plays a role in the control of ongoing saccades. Suzuki et al. [1981] reported that Purkinje cell activities related to smooth-pursuit eye movements were recorded in the posterior vermis. In the voluntary OKN of the present patient with Arnold-Chiari malformation, saccadic pursuit and dysmetria for the target catch were noted. These results suggest that the irregularity of wave form in voluntary OKN is due to disturbance of the posterior vermis. Kawasaki et al. [1981] reported that the slow phase of OKN velocity was in a lower range than normal at the higher OKN stimulus velocities in cats with hemicerebellectomy inclusive of the flocculus. In our present case, in which dysfunction of the flocculus was suggested, the eye speed in the slow phase in voluntary OKN was decreased at high cylinder speed, as reported by Kawasaki et al. [1981]. The eye speed of the slow phase in reflexive OKN was decreased at all cylinder speeds. Therefore, these results suggest that the flocculus contributes to reflexive OKN. In the case indicating atrophy of the brain stem and cerebellum, both OKN were disturbed. The characteristics of OKN in cerebellar disorders differ according to the site of the lesion. These features were clearly demonstrated by qualitative and quantitative tests.

References

Braak, J.W.G. Ter: Untersuchungen über optokinetischen Nystagmus. Arch. Neerl. Physiol. *21:* 309–376 (1936).

Hishida, N.: Abnormal optokinetic nystagmus in cerebellar disturbance. Pract. Otol., Kyoto *77:* suppl. 1, pp. 312–339 (1984).

Kase, M.; Miller, D.C.; Noda, H.: Discharges of Purkinje cells and mossy fibers in cerebellar vermis of the monkey during saccadic eye movements and fixation. J. Physiol., Lond. *300:* 539–555 (1980).

Kawasaki, T.; Kato, I.; Sato, Y.; Mizukoshi, K.: The brain-stem projection to the cerebellar flocculus relevant to optokinetic response in cats. Ann. N.Y. Acad. Sci. *374:* 455–464 (1981).

Suzuki, D.A.; Noda, H.; Kase, M.: Visual and pursuit eye movement-related activity in posterior vermis of monkey cerebellum. J. Neurophysiol. *46:* 1120–1139 (1981).

Tokita, T.; Suzuki, T.; Hibi, T.; Tomita, T.: A quantitative test of optokinetic nystagmus and its data processing by computer. Acta oto-lar., suppl. 330, pp. 159–168 (1975).

Tokita, T.; Suzuki, T.; Hishida, N.; Yanagida, M.: Examination of optokinetic nystagmus in relation to target movement. Adv. Oto-Rhino-Laryng., vol. 30, pp. 83–87 (Karger, Basel 1983).

K. Mizuta, MD, Department of Otorhinolaryngology,
Gifu University School of Medicine, Gifu 500 (Japan)

Adv. Oto-Rhino-Laryng., vol. 42, pp. 210–212 (Karger, Basel 1988)

Otoneurological Symptomatology in Lyme Disease

H. Krejcova, M. Bojar, J. Jerabek, J. Tomas, J. Jirous

Department of Neurology, Pediatric Faculty, Charles University,
Prague, Czechoslovakia

Introduction

An increasing number of reports concerning Lyme disease (LD) caused by the spirochaete *Borrelia burgdorferi* infection lack reference to otoneurological symptomatology. Reik et al. [1979] and Steere et al. [1983] mentioned the presence of neurologic abnormalities in their papers which included cerebellar ataxia and facial palsy. Additional otolaryngologic manifestation included otalgia, sore throat or dizziness in the early course of the disease. We did not find any paper dealing with vestibular symptomatology in LD.

Materials and Methods

Sixteen subjects out of the total amount of 39 patients suffering from LD revealed neuro-otological symptomatology. This group consisted of 5 men and 11 women aged 18–67 years. All underwent neurologic and otolaryngologic examination including ENG, EEG, EMG, BAEP, electrogustometry and tympanometry, CSF analysis and serological examination.

Results

The symptoms of vertigo and instability with or without hypacusis or tinnitus even before the occurrence of other neurologic symptomatology were observed in 6 patients. Spontaneous nystagmus was found in 2 cases, gaze nystagmus in 3 and positional in one. Caloric and rotational hyperresponsiveness appeared in one patient, hypoexcitability was found also in one. Vestibular areflexia was present in 4 patients, in 3 of them bilaterally, in one unilaterally. Directional preponderance (DP) was observed in 5 patients, in all of them of central origin. A marked dysrhythmia of the caloric and rotational response observed during repeated stimulation was present in 2 subjects. An impaired optokinetic response was found in 3 patients, at all stimulation frequencies, in the fourth patient it was influenced by the DP. The saccades were abnormal in 7 patients, in 6 of them there was simultaneous impairment of the eye tracking movements. The fixation-suppression test was abnormal in 5 patients bilaterally. Summarizing all the results of vestibular examination we found in one case the evidence of peripheral and in 12 patients of central type of vestibular abnormality.

Cochlear portion of the VIIIth nerve was impaired in 7 cases. In 4 of them there was symmetrical and in one asymmetrical perceptive hypacusis, normalized in later course of the disease. In 5 patients BAEP revealed prolonged latency of the IIIrd to Vth wave and asymmetry of amplitudes as a sign of brain stem disorder, again normalized within several months. Facial nerve palsy was present in 7 patients, in 4 bilaterally, in the other 3 unilaterally. The topical lesion of the VIIth nerve revealed in 6 patients genicular or suprastapedial and in one patient suprachordal type of involvement. The simultaneous impairment of both portions of VIIIth and of facial nerve was ascertained in 4 patients.

All patients of the examined group revealed pathological neurological findings: in 4 patients we found polyradiculoneuritic syndrome accompanied by a lesion of the VIIth and VIIIth nerves in 3 of them. Eight patients showed encephalomyelopolyradiculoneuritic involvement; in 2 of them also the distal cranial nerves were affected, in 6 of them the CNS involvement was complicated by VIIIth nerve lesion. Three patients showed signs of encephalitis with simultaneous involvement of the VIIIth nerve. One patient suffered from cranial polyneuritis including the VIIIth nerve lesion. In patients with CNS involvement of the brain stem or cerebral hemispheres the EEG showed diffuse abnormality in the former and focal temporal lesion in the latter ones.

Summarizing pathological findings in our patients, we proved vestibular abnormality in 81, hearing abnormality in 44, various neurological findings in 94 and facial palsy in 50% of patients.

Discussion

Later symptoms of LD developing after the skin and nonspecific symptoms are of most interest to the neurologist and otoneurologist. The aim of our paper is to accentuate occurrence of subjective or objective otoneurologic symptoms in 81% of patients with neurologic symptomatology and to show that in 38% of them it was as the first symptom of the whole clinical symptomatology. The prevalence of central type of vestibular finding suggests a more extensive involvement of the VIIIth nerve affecting not only the region of vestibular nuclei but also their pathways in the brain stem and cerebellum. In 44% of our patients with LD the lesion of the cochlear part of the VIIIth nerve fully confirms the necessity of complex otoneurologic examination in early diagnostics and treatment. The follow-up period of the patients revealed transient incidence of vestibular symptomatology in some affected persons, while in others it persisted with variable clinical pattern. This observation may confirm the possible role of reinfection or reactivation in some cases of chronic progressive form of LD. Further course of LD can be influenced by immunogenetic factors and aberrant HLA-DR expression which can provoke an autoimmune disease initiated by spirochaete infection.

References

Glasscock, M.E.; Pensak, M.L.; Gulya, A.J.; Baker, D.C.: Lyme disease. A cause of bilateral facial paralysis. Archs Otolar. *111:* 47–49 (1985).
Reik, L.; Steere, A.C.; Bartenhagen, N.H.: Neurologic abnormalities of Lyme disease. Medicine *58:* 281–294 (1979).
Steere, A.C.; Bartenhagen, N.W.; Craft, J.E.: The early clinical manifestations of Lyme disease. Ann. intern. Med. *99:* 76–82 (1983).

Prof. Dr. H. Krejcova, DSc, Department of Neurology, Pediatric Faculty, V uvalu 84, 150 18 Prague 5-Motol (Czechoslovakia)

Adv. Oto-Rhino-Laryng., vol. 42, pp. 213–216 (Karger, Basel 1988)

Dementia and Eye Movements

Setsuko Takemori[a], *Masayoshi Ida*[b,1]

[a]Neurotology and [b]Neurology, Toranomon Hospital and Okinaka Memorial Institute for Medical Research, Toranomon, Minato-ku, Tokyo, Japan

The population of elderly people is increasing as the periods of life are prolonged; therefore, people with dementia are going to increase. In cases of dementia, disturbance of understanding is the most evident sign, and their behaviors are very simple and childish.

There are many kinds of dementia: cerebral lesions, cortical dementia, subcortical dementia, etc. Cortical dementia, especially Alzheimer's type of dementia, and dementia caused by cerebral vascular lesions have been studied.

Subjects

Eighteen cases of dementia with cerebral lesions have been studied.

	Cases
Etiology	
Angiogenic	7
Alzheimer's type	4
Post meningitis	3
Brain metastasis	3
Postoperative (cerebral tumor)	1
Sex	
Male	12
Female	6

[1] We would like to express our thanks to Mrs. H. Moriyama for her technical assistance.

	Cases
Age	
31–40	1
41–50	2
51–60	3
61–70	6
71–80	6

Methods

Examinations of Eye Movements

Spontaneous nystagmus, gaze nystagmus, positional and positioning nystagmus were observed under the Frenzel glasses and they were recorded by electronystagmography (ENG). Horizontal and vertical eye movements were simultaneously recorded by silver plate electrodes, or by scleral search coils. Pursuit, optokinetic nystagmus (OKN), caloric nystagmus and visual suppression were examined and recorded by ENG.

Pursuit. A round target of 1 cm diameter moved circularly with the visual angle of 30° and with the cycle of 0.25 Hz.

Optokinetic Nystagmus. OKN was evoked by rotating a drum of 180 cm diameter with 12 black stripes inside and this drum was driven electroautomatically. The drum was accelerated by 4 °/s^2 from 0 to 150 °/s and decelerated from 150 to 0 °/s.

OKN was recorded by the paper speed of 1 mm/s, and it was shown as patterns (OKN patterns, OKP). Right and left OKP were examined.

Caloric Test and Visual Suppression. 20 ml of water at 5 °C was irrigated into the external auditory canal for 20 s. Caloric nystagmus was recorded by ENG and the slow phase velocity of caloric nystagmus was measured to compare the responses of the right and left ears. Visual suppression was also measured.

Evaluation of Dementia

A screening test of mental disorders was used. This examination was very similar to the DMS III of the USA [1]. The score of 0–10 indicated the possibility of dementia; 10–15 was borderline and dementia suspected, 15–20 was normal.

Results and Conclusion

Disturbance of eye movements were seen in all cases of dementia.

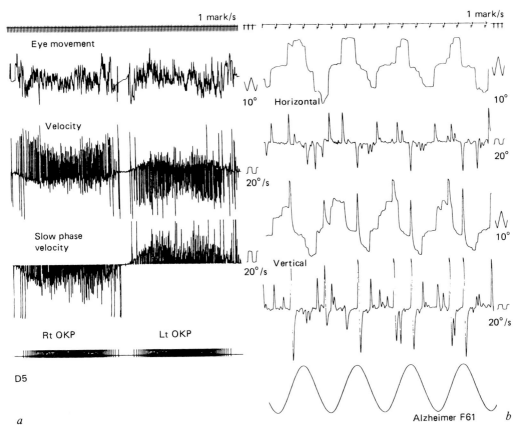

Fig. 1. A 61-year-old female with Alzheimer's type of dementia. *a* OKN patterns. The slow phase velocity and the frequency of OKN patterns are within normal limits. *b* Pursuit eye movements. Both horizontal and vertical eye movements show ataxic and saccadic pursuits.

Alzheimer Type

There was no gaze or spontaneous nystagmus. Very mild vertical positioning nystagmus was seen as well as saccadic and ataxic pursuit. OKN, caloric nystagmus and visual suppression was normal (fig. 1).

Multiple Infarct Dementia

Disturbance of eye movements increased with the severing of the mental disorders. Pursuit eye movements were impaired in all cerebral lesions;

however, disturbance of pursuit was not strong in temporal lobe lesions. OKN showed asymmetry. The OKN to the lesion side was better than the OKN to the contralateral side. OKN to the ipsilateral side was normal, and OKN to the contralateral side was slightly impaired. This is the typical finding of OKN in cerebral lesions. In the lower parietal lobe lesions, OKN to the ipsilateral side was impaired, and it was better than the OKN to the contralateral side. Caloric nystagmus showed no asymmetry. Visual suppression was normal in cases of frontal, temporal, upper parietal lobe and occipital lobe lesion. It was greatly impaired in cases with lower parietal lobe lesions [2, 3]. There were no voluntary eye movements in the most severe cases. Thus, eye movement disturbance was related to the involvement of lower parietal lobe lesions.

References

1 American Psychiatric Association: Diagnostic and statistical manual of mental disorders; 3rd ed. (Am. Psychiatric Association, Washington 1980).
2 Bálint, R.: Sehlähmung des 'Schauens', optische Ataxie, räumliche Störung der Aufmerksamkeit. Mschr. Psychiat. Neurol. *25:* 51–81 (1909).
3 Takemori, S.; Ishikawa, M.; Yamada, S.: Cerebral control of eye movements. ORL *43:* 262–273 (1981).

Dr. Setsuko Takemori, Neurotology, Toranomon Hospital, 2–2–2 Toranomon, Minato-ku, Tokyo 105 (Japan)

Adv. Oto-Rhino-Laryng., vol. 42, pp. 217–218 (Karger, Basel 1988)

Familial Head Movement Dependent Oscillopsia

W.I.M. Verhagen[a], *P.L.M. Huygen*[b]

[a]Department of Neurology, Canisius-Wilhelmina Hospital; [b]ENT Department, Radboud University Hospital, Nijmegen, The Netherlands

Some patients report the symptom of illusory movements of the visual world during head movements only, which is known as head-movement-dependent oscillopsia (HMDO). This may be due to peripheral vestibular, brain stem or cerebellar disorders [for review, ref. 1]. Two families are reported with HMDO due to peripheral vestibular dysfunction.

In the first family 2 brothers and a sister had HMDO as long as they could remember. They also mentioned blurred vision, and broad-based gait during walking in the dark. There was no hearing loss. They had no history of other neurologic or otologic disorders, nor of the use of neuro-ototoxic drugs. The rest of the family history was negative. All showed vestibular areflexia. Audiograms were normal. Ocular motor tests were normal (smooth pursuit, saccades and optokinetic nystagmus) except for the absence of optokinetic afternystagmus. Petrosum X-ray films, brain computer-assisted tomography and extensive laboratory studies were normal. The pedigree suggests an autosomal recessive mode of inheritance. The conclusion was that these patients probably had a congenital vestibular areflexia.

In the second family several members mentioned HMDO at about 40 years of age. Several years later all affected persons had a progressive sensorineural hearing loss as was established by audiograms. They had no nausea and vomiting. There was no history of other neurologic and otologic disorders, nor of the use of neuro-ototoxic drugs. Family history revealed at least 4 cases; we examined 2 of them. They had vestibular areflexia combined with progressive sensorineural hearing loss. Petrosum X-ray films, brain CT scans and laboratory tests were normal. Brain stem auditory responses showed normal I–V, I–III, and III–V interlatency times. We suggest that the patients in this family suffer from a familial progressive vestibulocochlear disorder of the inner ear. The pedigree revealed an autosomal dominant mode of inheritance.

The first family has a dysfunction that has not been reported before [2]. There are several hereditary disorders with sensorineural hearing loss without other abnormalities [3]. Vestibular tests were not performed or normal in these disorders, so the disorder in the second family also seems to be a new clinical entity.

References

1   Hess, K.; Gresty, M.; Leech, J.: Clinical and theoretical aspects of head movement dependent oscillopsia (HMDO). J. Neurol. *219:* 151–157 (1978).
2   Verhagen, W.I.M.; Huygen, P.L.M.; Horstink, M.W.I.M.: Familial congenital vestibular areflexia. J. Neurol. Neurosurg. Psychiat. *50:* 933–935 (1987).
3   Konigsmark, B.W.; Gorlin, R.J.: Genetic and metabolic deafness (Saunders, Philadelphia 1976).

Dr. W.I.M. Verhagen, Department of Neurology, Canisius-Wilhelmina Hospital, St. Annastraat 289, NL-6525 GS Nijmegen (The Netherlands)

Adv. Oto-Rhino-Laryng., vol. 42, pp. 219–223 (Karger, Basel 1988)

Vestibular Involvement in Spasmodic Torticollis: An Old Hypothesis with New Data from Otolith Testing

Shirley G. Diamond, Charles H. Markham, Robert W. Baloh

Department of Neurology, UCLA School of Medicine, Los Angeles, Calif., USA

Spasmodic torticollis is a focal dystonic movement disorder character-ized by involuntary turning of the neck by forceful spasms. The chin may be rotated to one side or the other, or the head pulled forward or backward.

The cause of spasmodic torticollis is unknown. It is generally thought to involve the extrapyramidal or midbrain structures, but the findings in postmortem examinations have not been consistent. From time to time, the suggestion has been made that the vestibular system may be involved. Gowers [1], in 1893, proposed that torticollis might be due to 'aural maladies'. In 1943, Patterson and Little [2] published a comprehensive review of the torticollis literature to that time, and concluded that the vestibular pathways were important, and that the otolith system must be involved because symptoms were eased when patients assumed a supine position.

Torticollis patients have been reported to have more spontaneous nystagmus and abnormal calorics than expected. EMG studies of torticollis patients report that when the ear ipsilateral to the affected side of the neck is irrigated with cold water, the tonic neck muscle activity increases, and that cold water irrigation in the contralateral ear lessens or abolishes involuntary contractions. Neck muscles in normal subjects are not influenced by this stimulation. A recent retrospective study of vestibular function in patients with spasmodic torticollis by Bronstein and Rudge [3] found a high incidence of spontaneous nystagmus and caloric abnormalities.

Having developed in our laboratory a test of otolith function, ocular counterrolling (OCR), it was possible to examine the question of whether this otolith reflex is affected in spasmodic torticollis.

Subjects were strapped into a tilting chair controlled by an Apple IIe computer. The centers of the pupils were aligned horizontally, and the head positioned and stabilized by a bite bar. Subjects were rotated at a constant velocity of 3 °/s to 90° right ear down, held there for a few seconds, rolled to 90° left ear down, and then returned to the starting position (trial I). Without stopping, the procedure was repeated (trial II). Acceleration and deceleration were 0.21 °/s², below semicircular canal thresholds. This test was performed in both naso-occipital (N-O) roll and also in earth-horizontal long axis or barbecue (BBQ) rotation, with the same protocol in both modes of rotation. Photographs of the upper face were taken at each 10° of rotation.

Measurements of OCR were made with a dual projector system linked to another Apple IIe computer, printer and plotter. The image of the counterrolled eye is rotated until it exactly superimposes the image of the eye in the control position. The extent of rotation that the image has to undergo to achieve perfect superimposition is the measure of torsion that the eye has undergone. Each eye is measured independently. This system is accurate to 0.1°.

The measurements were plotted on a form showing the mean OCR of normal subjects in the N-O rotations. OCR in normal subjects in BBQ rotation is very similar to responses in N-O roll.

We tested 8 patients with spasmodic torticollis, 2 men and 6 women, mean age 51 years. Three patients had chin deviation to the right, 3 to the left, one had anterocollis with some deviation to the left, and one was in almost perfect remission of 9 years' duration from severe torticollis to the left. They underwent testing in both N-O and BBQ rotations. Seven of the 8 patients also had ENG and caloric testing performed.

Results

All 8 patients had abnormal counterrolling. Figure 1 shows the N-O roll of a 42-year-old woman with torticollis to the right. Notably abnormal was the finding that at the extreme positions, the OCR reflex failed to be sustained, resulting in the eyes 'rolling' rather than counterrolling. This occurred in both directions of tilt. Her OCR also showed a lack of smoothness, particularly in trial II. Incidentally, the man who was in remission showed OCR which was mildly but definitely abnormal. He too showed the rolling phenomenon.

Figure 2 summarizes the abnormalities found in our torticollis patients. In general, we can say that the defects were apparent in N-O and BBQ modes

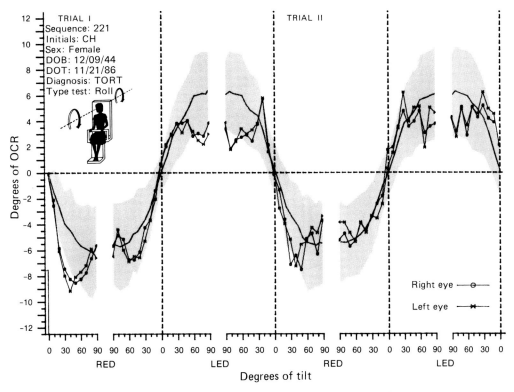

Fig. 1. Typical spasmodic torticollis patient, with chin deviation to right, showed rolling rather than counterrolling in the regions near 90° tilt. This failure to sustain OCR in the extreme positions was seen previously only in patients with brain stem compression. Mean responses of normal subjects are shown by smooth line.

about equally. In the BBQ rotations the ipsilateral tilts were more abnormal than the contralateral. The most dramatic finding was the presence of rolling, with 100% of patients showing this in ipsilateral BBQ tilt and 88% in ipsilateral N-O roll.

In ENG testing performed on 7 patients, 5 or 71% had spontaneous vestibular nystagmus in the sitting position with eyes open in the dark. This was to the ipsilateral side in 2 cases and to the contralateral in 3. With caloric stimulation, 3 of these 5 patients demonstrated preponderances in the same direction as their spontaneous vestibular nystagmus.

Although OCR function was clearly disturbed in our spasmodic torticollis patients, the types of abnormalities differed from those that we observed in other disorders [4, 5]. Because our past studies have shown rolling

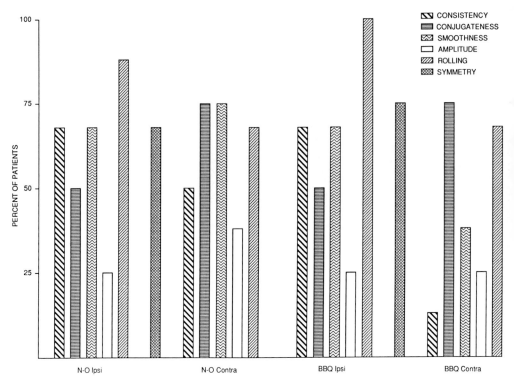

Fig. 2. Of the several OCR defects seen in spasmodic torticollis, the most prevalent was rolling, present in 100% in BBQ ipsi and 88% in N–O ipsi rotations. BBQ and N–O modes were equally abnormal. Ipsilateral tilts revealed a few more defects than contralateral.

primarily in patients with known brain stem difficulties [6], the present occurrence of this phenomenon leads us to infer that the disorder in spasmodic torticollis lies in central vestibular connections and is a manifestation of the disruption of brain stem pathwyas. The directional preponderance found with caloric stimulation suggests a vestibular imbalance without localizing the origin.

We conclude that otolith function is definitely abnormal in patients with spasmodic torticollis. Although a great deal of evidence implicates the vestibular system in this disorder, it is not at all clear whether the vestibular role is a primary, etiologic one or a secondary effect stemming either from the chronically tipped otoliths or from asymmetric inputs from neck afferents to vestibular nuclei.

References

1   Gowers, W.R.: A manual of diseases of the nervous system, vol. 2, pp. 662–663 (Blakiston, Philadelphia 1893).
2   Patterson, R.M.; Little, S.C.: Spasmodic torticollis. J. nerv. ment. Dis. *98:* 571–599 (1943).
3   Bronstein, A.M.; Rudge, P.: Vestibular involvement in spasmodic torticollis. J. Neurol. Neurosurg. Psychiat. *49:* 290–295 (1986).
4   Diamond, S.G.; Markham, C.H.: Ocular counterrolling as an indicator of vestibular otolith function. Neurology *33:* 1460–1469 (1983).
5   Markham, C.H.; Diamond, S.G.; Ito, J.: Utricular dysfunction in benign paroxysmal positional vertigo; in Graham, Kemink, The vestibular system: neurophysiologic and clinical research, chap. 32, pp. 275–283 (Raven Press, New York 1987).
6   Markham, C.H.; Diamond, S.G.: Distinctive ocular counterrolling disruption caused by brainstem compression; in Kunze et al., Clinical problems of brainstem disorders (Thieme, Stuttgart 1986).

Shirley G. Diamond, Department of Neurology, UCLA School of Medicine,
Los Angeles, CA 90024–1769 (USA)

Adv. Oto-Rhino Laryng., vol. 42, pp. 224–228 (Karger, Basel 1988)

The Effect of Serotonin on the Pontine Pause Neurons in the Cat

Nobuhiko Furuya, Hidemichi Ashikawa, Takao Yabe, Jun-Ichi Suzuki

Department of Otolaryngology, Teikyo University School of Medicine, Itabashi-ku, Tokyo, Japan

Most of the detailed analyses of vestibular nystagmus have been carried out in the cat by examination of various types of brain stem neurons [2, 3, 6–9, 12]. Although the neural organization of vestibular nystagmus has recently been well analyzed, there have been few systematic studies of the transmitter of these nystagmus-related neurons [12]. Pause neurons (PN), which are clustered in the pontine raphe nuclei, are critical for the production of voluntary and involuntary saccadic eye movement. They exhibit a tonic discharge when the eyes are not moving or during slow eye movements, and abruptly stop firing just before and during rapid eye movements. The raphe region of the brain stem contains the neurons which produce serotonin (5-HT), and also has 5-HT-sensitive receptor sites, probably the terminals of the 5-HT-axon collaterals [1]. The neurons which control the pause neuronal activity are still not known, although if the nature of the neurotransmitter were to be clarified, it should be easy to find the higher neurons responsible. The present experiment was designed in order to find a candidate neurotransmitter which would cause the abrupt stoppage of PN firing during vestibular nystagmus.

Eighteen adult cats were anesthetized with ether and mounted in a stereotaxic apparatus on a turntable. Bipolar stimulation electrodes were placed in the bilateral middle ear for vestibular nerve stimulation. The right abducens and medial rectus nerves were detached from their respective innervating muscles and mounted on fine Ag-AgCl hook electrodes for the monitoring of nystagmus (fig. 1a). Three-barrelled glass microelectrodes, filled with 3 M KCl, 0.05 M 5-hydroxytryptamine (pH 3.5), 3 M L-glutamate

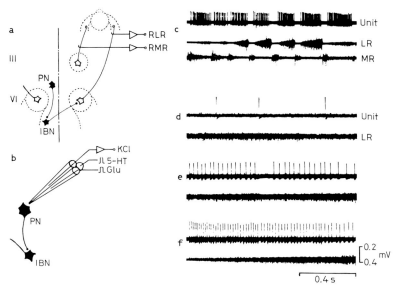

Fig. 1. Schematic diagram of experimental conditions (*a, b*) and physiological features of a pause neuron (PN) during vestibular nystagmus (*b–d*). *a* Simultaneous recordings of the extracellular PN spike discharge and that of the abducens (RLR) and the medial rectus (RMR) nerve. III, IV and IBN: IIIrd and VIth nuclei and inhibitory burst neuron, respectively. *b* Unit recording with three-barrelled glass microelectrode which was filled with 3 *M* KCl for unit recording, and 5-hydroxytryptamine and glutamate for drug application. *c–f* Recordings from the same neuron, showing the typical discharge pattern of PN in *c*. Iontophoretically administered 5-HT using 60 nA (*d*) and glutamate using 80 nA (*f*). *d* is the control recording for *d* and *f*.

(pH 8.5) or 0.01 *M* methysergide (pH 7.0) were used for recording and drug application (fig. 1b). Glutamate was iontophoretically injected as anion, and methysergide and 5-HT were administered as cations. The occipital bone was removed and the vermal part of cerebellum was aspirated to expose the fourth ventricle. The animals were also maintained in a pain-free condition by infiltrating 0.5% lidocaine with epinephrine into the wound sites and pressure points. All recordings were taken with the cats in an alert condition following upper cervical cord transection and under artificial respiration. The effectiveness of the local anesthetic in controlling pain was carefully checked by observing blood pressure, heart rate, pulse pressure and pupillary size [3].

Simultaneous recordings of the extracellular PN spike discharge, and of the abducens and the medial rectus nerves, were made. If the neurons exhibited a tonic discharge during the slow phase of nystagmus and a pause in discharge during the quick phase of nystagmus (PN behavior), they were then subjected to further study. Twenty-eight neurons were identified as PN under the present criteria. One of these is shown in figure 1. This neuron showed a clear pause at the quick-phase discharges of the abducens or medial rectus nerves (fig. 1c). d, e and f are unit recordings showing the effects of topical administration of 5-HT (d) and glutamate (f). The tonic discharges of PN were consistently suppressed by 5-HT application (fig. 1d), but their unit activities were facilitated by iontophoretic administration of glutamate (fig. 1f). Iontophoretically administered serotonin suppressed 18 out of 28 PN investigated. There was considerable variation in the sensitivity of individual PN to serotonin, the threshold ranging from 40 nA to a current intensity greater than 200 nA. The action appeared immediately after the onset of the injection current, but considerable variations were observed in the time course of the response after cessation of the current. Usually the effects lasted 50–200 ms.

The relationship between the iontophoretic current used for injection of serotonin and the resulting suppression of spike discharges was investigated. The plateau level of the dose-response curve varied from unit to unit. As might be expected from the fading response to continued administration of serotonin, the effectiveness of subsequent doses depended on the previous dose. The dose-response curve is summarized in fig. 2a. In order to normalize the variations of spontaneous discharge in individual PN, pretreatment level of discharge was considered as 100%. The data were obtained from 8 neurons, which showed a similar threshold ranging from 40 to 50 nA.

In order to make sure that these suppressions were caused by serotonin, systemic injection of methysergide, a specific serotonin blocker, was applied. Another typical baseline recording of PN and ocular nerve potentials during manual rotation of the turntable is shown in figure 2b. The neuron, upon administration of serotonin showing current at 150 nA, showed strong suppression of firing activity (fig. 2c.) The animal then received methysergide (1 mg/kg i.v.) and, after 20 min, the neuron was treated with serotonin using the same current as before (fig. 2c). This time, spontaneous discharge of the neuron was not suppressed, and the rhythmic pause pattern also recovered. The effect of methysergide was observed within 15 min and lasted as long as 60 min. These effects were consistently observed in 12 treated neurons.

Serotonin produces both excitation and inhibition, and these effects are thought to be mediated by two different receptors [13, 15]. Although not conclusively proven, several studies have suggested that methysergide blocks

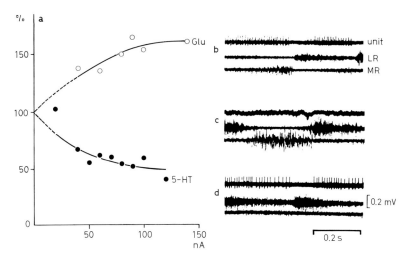

Fig. 2. The influences of glutamate, 5-HT and methysergide on PN. *a* Dose-response curve of serotonin and glutamate summarized from eight PN. Ordinate represents mean spike frequency expressed as a percentage of the control value with the backing current and the abscissa iontophoretic currents (nA) used to inject these chemicals. Glu = Glutamate. *b–d* The effect of systemic application of methysergide. Baseline recording of PN is shown in *b*. Iontophoretically applied 5-HT (150 nA) caused potent inhibition of the PN (*c*), but this effect was suppressed by intravenous application of methysergide (1 mg/kg).

only excitatory serotonin receptors [5, 10, 11]. The present data revealed that PN showed inhibition of their spike discharges by serotonin, and that not only the spike discharges but also the rhythmical pause patterns were restored by methysergide. The fact that topical application of serotonin to PN caused suppression of spike discharges confirmed the results of recent studies that the serotonergic terminals on the raphe serotonergic neurons appear to be inhibitory. However, the phenomenon of the recovered pause pattern after methysergide administration needs further explanation. It is possible to explain these phenomena by supposing that PN have at least two different types of inhibitory receptors (a 5-HT type and another type), i.e. that PN receive inhibitory synaptic terminals (non-5-HT) from higher neurons which cause a pause pattern in the PN, and that they also receive other inhibitory synaptic terminals from adjacent inhibitory neurons, which bear the excitatory serotonin receptor.

At the beginning of this study, we simply speculated that serotonin would cause a pause reaction in PN. However, this speculation now seems unlikely, because PN showed clear pause behavior after the administration of methysergide. If methysergide blocks the inhibitory serotonin receptors, then PN should show tonic discharges instead of a pause pattern. The present findings strongly suggest that pause neurons receive two inhibitory pathways, one consisting of impulses from higher serotonergic neurons and the other consisting of nonserotonergic neurons. The former neurons support the baseline activity of PN, while the latter might be important for rhythm formation.

References

1 Aghajanian, G.K.; Haigler, H.J.: Direct and indirect actions of LSD, serotonin and related compounds on serotonin-containing neurons; in Barchas, Usdin, Serotonin and behavior, p. 615 (Academic Press, New York 1973).
2 Curthoys, I.S.; Nakao, S.; Markham, C.H.: Cat medial pontine reticular neurons related to vestibular nystagmus. Firing pattern, location and projection. Brain Res. *222:* 75–94 (1981).
3 Furuya, N.; Markham, C.H.: Direct inhibitory synaptic linkage of pause neurons with burst inhibitory neurons. Brain Res. *245:* 139–143 (1982).
4 Haigler, H.J.; Aghajanian, G.K.: Lysergic acid diethylamide and serotonin. A comparison of effects on serotonergic neurons and neurons receiving a serotonergic input. J. Pharmac. exp. Ther. *188:* 688–699 (1974).
5 Haigler, H.J.; Aghajanian, G.K.: Peripheral serotonin antagonists. Failure to antagonize serotonin in brain areas receiving a prominent serotonergic input. J. neural. Transm. *35:* 257–273 (1974).
6 Highstein, S.M.; Baker, R.: Excitatory termination of abducens internuclear neurons on medial rectus motoneurons. Relationship to syndrome of internuclear ophthalmoplegia. J. Neurophysiol. *41:* 1647–1661 (1978).
7 Hikosaka, O.; Maeda, M.; Nakao, S.; Shimazu, H.; Shinoda, Y.: Presynaptic impulses in the abducens nucleus and their relation to postsynaptic potentials in motoneurons during vestibular nystagmus. Exp. Brain Res. *27:* 355–376 (1977).
8 Maeda, M.; Shimazu, H.; Shinoda, Y.: Nature of synaptic events in cat abducens motoneurons at slow and quick phase of vestibular nystagmus. J. Neurophysiol. *35:* 279–296 (1972).
9 Nakao, S.; Sasaki, S.: Firing pattern of interneurons in the abducens nucleus related to vestibular nystagmus in the cat. Brain Res. *144:* 389–394 (1978).
10 Peroutka, S.J.; Lebovitz, R.M.; Snyder, S.H.: Two distinct central serotonin receptors with different physiologic functions. Sci. *212:* 827–830 (1981).
11 Roberts, M.H.T.; Stranghan, D.W.: Excitation and depression of cortical neurons by 5-hydroxytryptamine. J. Physiol., Lond. *193:* 269–294 (1967).
12 Baloh, R.W.; Markham, C.H.; Furuya, N.: Inhibition of pontine omnipauser neurons in the cat by 5-hydroxytryptophan. Expl. Neurol. *76:* 586–593 (1982).

Nobuhiko Furuya, MD, Department of Otolaryngology, Teikyo University
School of Medicine, Kaga 2-11-1, Itabashi-ku, Tokyo 173 (Japan)

Adv. Oto-Rhino Laryng., vol. 42, pp. 229–233 (Karger, Basel 1988)

The Role of NMDA and Non-NMDA Receptors in the Central Vestibular Synaptic Transmission

Thomas Knöpfel, Norbert Dieringer

Brain Research Institute, University of Zürich, Zürich, Switzerland

Excitatory amino acids (e.g. glutamate, aspartate and homocysteate) are thought to mediate synaptic transmission at many synapses in the central nervous system. Pharmacological investigations have shown that these transmitter candidates interact with different receptors [Watkins, 1981] among which the N-methyl-*D*-aspartate (NMDA) type has attracted particular attention. In comparison with non-NMDA types of excitatory amino acid receptors, the activation of NMDA receptors results in some rather unconventional effects on membrane properties. Thus, NMDA induces an inward membrane current, characterized by a region of negative slope conductance [Mayer and Westbrook, 1984]. As a consequence of this property NMDA can enhance the efficacy of subsequent converging synaptic inputs. Recent studies suggested an involvement of NMDA receptors in synaptic plasticity such as long-term potentiation [Collingridge et al., 1983] and ocular dominance shift induced by monocular deprivation [Kleinschmidt et al., 1986].

In view of the known vestibular synaptic plasticity, we studied the role of NMDA receptors in this system. The vestibular system of the frog has been extensively studied anatomically (Grofova and Corvaja, 1972; Matesz, 1979], physiologically [Precht, 1976] and pharmacologically [Cochran et al., 1987; Knöpfel, 1987]. The brain stem commissural system connects the bilateral vestibular nuclei through mainly excitatory pathways involving NMDA receptors.

The brain stem of either intact or hemilabyrinthectomized (HL) frogs (*Rana temporaria*) was isolated and kept in vitro [Cochran et al., 1987; Knöpfel, 1987]. Bipolar stimulating electrodes were placed on the distal end of the VIIIth nerve(s). Vestibular afferent field potentials in the vestibular nucleus and vestibular afferent excitatory postsynaptic potentials (EPSPs) of

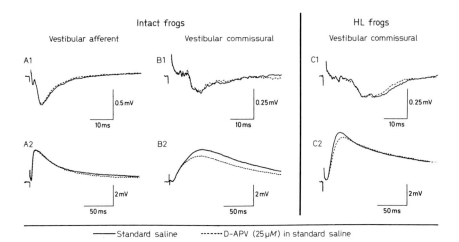

Fig. 1. Effects of the NMDA antagonist D-APV on potentials in the vestibular nuclear complex of intact and hemilabyrinthectomized (HL) frogs. A1–C1: Averaged (n = 16) field potentials. A2–C2: Averaged (n = 8) EPSPs. Vestibular afferents were activated by electrical stimulation of the VIIIth nerve on the ipsilateral side. Commissural inputs were evoked on the contralateral side (intact side in HL frogs). Continuous lines and dotted lines show potentials recorded in standard solution and in D-APV-containing solution, respectively.

central vestibular neurons were evoked by electrical stimulation of the ipsilateral VIIIth nerve. Vestibular commissural field potentials and commissural EPSPs were evoked by stimulation of the contralateral VIIIth nerve. During extra- and intracellular recordings, the preparation was continuously superfused with frog Ringer which always contained 1 mM Mg^{2+}. This solution could be exchanged for a superfusion fluid that contained the selective NMDA antagonist D-2-amino-5-phosphonovaleric acid [Davies et al., 1981] (D-APV. 25 µM in Ringer). Averages of field and synaptic potentials from either side, recorded in each of the two solutions, were compared in respect of their sensitivity to D-APV allowing the contribution of NMDA receptors to these potentials to be assessed.

The shape of vestibular afferent field potentials and EPSPs was not affected by D-APV (fig. 1 A1–A2). However, these potentials were abolished by the unspecific excitatory amino acid antagonist kynurenic acid [Cochran et al., 1987], indicating that the afferent vestibular excitation is mediated through non-NMDA synaptic receptors. Commissural EPSPs differ in their pharmacological sensitivities from vestibular afferent EPSPs in that they exhibit a delayed D-APV-sensitive component [Knöpfel, 1986a; Cochran et al., 1987] (fig. 1 B2). Interestingly, such a component is not detected in the concomitant field potential (fig. 1 B1). This discrepancy might be explained by evidence suggesting that NMDA receptors are tonically activated [Knöpfel, 1986a]. As a consequence of this persistent activation of receptors with specific properties, the effective membrane input resistance increases with the result that the efficacy of non-NMDA receptor-mediated commissural inputs is enhanced [Knöpfel, 1986b]. Such a modulatory influence of NMDA receptors on the synaptic efficacy of commissural and other converging inputs appears to be of particular interest in the context of short-term and long-term adaptations of the gain of vestibular reflexes [Dieringer and Precht, 1979; Galiana et al., 1984].

NMDA receptors could for instance be involved in the increase of the synaptic efficacy of vestibular commissural fibers on the lesioned side of chronic HL frogs [Dieringer and Precht, 1979]. We tested this possibility. As in controls, in chronic (more than 6 weeks) HL animals, commissurally evoked EPSPs (fig. 1 C2) but not field potentials (fig. 1 C1) exhibited an NMDA receptor-mediated component. D-APV reduced the amplitude of EPSPs to an amount that was positively related with the time to peak of EPSP. Thus, in intact animals the fast rising vestibular afferent EPSPs were not significantly affected but the more slowly rising commissural EPSPs were remarkably D-APV sensitive (fig. 2). In chronic HL animals the D-APV sensitive component of commissural EPSPs decreased with the decrease in their time to peak (fig. 2). EPSPs with similar shape parameters were similarly affected by D-APV irrespective of their recording in HL or in control frogs. Since the changes in the mean shape parameters of commissural EPSPs in HL frogs are not correlated with an increased D-APV sensitivity (fig. 2), we conclude that the increased efficacy in chronic animals is not due to an enhanced activation of NMDA receptors. These results suggest, in accordance with previous investigations [Dieringer and Precht, 1979], morphological alterations (sprouting/dendritic shrinkage) in the partially deafferented vestibular nucleus as a more likely mechanism for the increase in synaptic efficacy. However, a trigger function of NMDA receptors for the processes leading to an increase in synaptic efficacy after HL cannot be excluded.

At present the physiological significance of the described NMDA receptor-mediated EPSP component remains unclear. These NMDA receptors are able to modulate the efficacy of dendritic inputs that converge temporally and spatially. In vivo such a convergence of coactivated inputs occurs as long

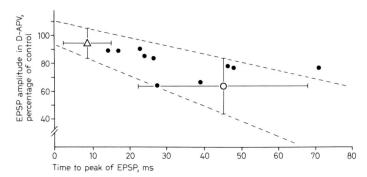

Fig. 2. D-APV sensitivity and time to peak of EPSPs in vestibular nuclear neurons of intact and chronic HL frogs. The amplitude of EPSPs recorded in D-APV-containing solution was expressed as percentage of the control amplitude obtained in standard saline and was plotted against the time to peak. Dots represent individual EPSPs recorded on the lesioned side of HL frogs. The triangle and circle represent mean values (± SD) of vestibular afferent and commissural EPSPs of controls, respectively. Note that the time to peak as well as the D-APV sensitivity of most of the commissural EPSPs of HL frogs lie between the mean values of afferent and commissural EPSPs of controls.

as head movements are not restricted to the horizontal plane. Thus, various combinations of dendritic convergences (canal-canal, canal-macular, etc.) could be gated and preferentially conducted to the soma depending on the degree of activation of NMDA receptors.

References

Cochran, S.L.; Kasik, P.; Precht, W.: Pharmacological aspects of excitatory synaptic transmission to second order vestibular neurons in the frog. Synapse *1:* 102–123 (1987).

Collingridge, G.L.; Kehl, S.J.; McLennan, H.: Excitatory amino acids in synaptic transmission in the Schaffer collateral-commissural pathway of the rat hippocampus. J. Physiol. *334:* 33–46 (1983).

Davies, J.; Francis, A.A.; Jones, A.W.; Watkins, J.C.: 2-Amino-5-phosphonovalerate (2-APV), a potent and selective antagonist of amino acid-induced and synaptic excitation. Neurosci. Lett. *21:* 77–81 (1981).

Dieringer, N.; Precht, W.: Mechanism of compensation for vestibular deficits in the frog. I. Modification of the excitatory commissural system. Exp. Brain Res. *36:* 311–328 (1979).

Galiana, H.L.; Flohr, H.; Melvill Jones, G.: A reevaluation of intervestibular nuclear coupling: its role in vestibular compensation. J. Neurophysiol. *51:* 242–259 (1984).

Grofova, I.; Corvaja, N.: Commissural projection from the nuclei of termination of the VIIIth cranial nerve in the toad. Brain Res. *42:* 189–195 (1972).

Kleinschmidt, A.; Bear, M.F.; Singer, W.: Effects of the NMDA-receptor antagonist APV on visual cortical plasticity in monocularly deprived kittens. Neurosci. Lett. *26:* suppl., p. S58 (1986).

Knöpfel, T.: How are NMDA receptors of central vestibular neurons activated? Experientia *42:* 638 (1986a).

Knöpfel, T.: Modulation of synaptic efficacy through NMDA-receptor activation. Neurosci. Lett. supp. *26:* S420 (1986b).

Knöpfel, T.: Evidence for N-methyl-*D*-aspartic acid-receptor-mediated modulation of the commissural input to central vestibular neurons of the frog. Brain Res. *426:* 212–224 (1987).

Matesz, C.: Central projections of the VIIIth cranial nerve in the frog. Neuroscience *4:* 2061–2071 (1979).

Mayer, M.; Westbrook, G.L.: Mixed-agonist action of excitatory amino acids on mouse spinal cord neurons under voltage clamp. J. Physiol. *354:* 29–53 (1984).

Precht, W.: Physiology of peripheral and central vestibular systems; in Llinas, Precht, Frog neurobiology, pp. 481–512 (Springer, Berlin 1976).

Watkins, J.C.: Pharmacology of excitatory amino acid neurotransmitters; in DeFeudis, Mandel, Amino acid neurotransmitters, pp. 205–212 (Raven Press, New York 1981).

Thomas Knöpfel, MD, Brain Research Institute, University of Zürich,
August Forelstrasse 1, CH-8029 Zürich (Switzerland)

Adv. Oto-Rhino-Laryng., vol. 42, pp. 234–237 (Karger, Basel 1988)

Is the Noradrenergic Neuron System in the Brain Stem Related to Motion Sickness in Rats?

N. Takeda[a], *M. Morita*[a], *T. Kubo*[a], *A. Yamatodani*[b], *H. Wada*[b], *T. Matsunaga*[a]

Department of [a]Otolaryngology and [b]Pharmacology II, Osaka University School of Medicine, Osaka, Japan

Introduction

Amphetamine is used clinically as an anti-motion sickness drug, and its efficacy in controlling acute experimental motion sickness in humans has been established [4, 10]. Rats also suffer from motion sickness when subjected to complex rotation, and pica can be used as an index of the extent of their motion sickness [7, 9]. Their motion sickness can also be prevented by administration of amphetamine [8]. Since amphetamine activates noradrenergic neuron system to increase release of noradrenaline from the nerve terminals, the noradrenergic neuron system in the brain is thought to be important in the development of motion sickness [10, 11]. But the exact role of noradrenaline in motion sickness is unknown.

Noradrenaline in the central nervous system is metabolized to 3-methoxy-4-hydroxyphenylglycol (MHPG), the production of which is directly related to the functional activity of the central noradrenergic neurons. Thus, change in the level of MHPG is a reliable indicator of the noradrenergic nervous activity in the brain.

In the present study, by measuring the contents of noradrenaline and its major metabolite, MHPG, we investigated the effects of rotational stimulation to produce motion sickness in rats on the activity of the noradrenergic neuron system in their brain stem.

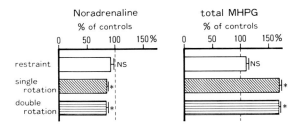

Fig. 1. Effects of restraint, and single and double rotations on the concentration of noradrenaline and total MHPG in the rat brain stem. Animals were sacrificed after restraint or rotation for 60 min. Columns and bars represent means ± SE for 10 animals as percentages of the mean values in control animals. *p<0.01 versus control value.

Materials and Methods

Male Wistar strain rats weighing about 150 g were divided into four experimental groups. The first group was placed in the restraining applicator and rotated about two parallel axes simultaneously (double rotation). The second group was placed in the applicator and rotated about one axis (single rotation). Measurement of kaolin intake as an index of motion sickness of rats showed that double rotation produced motion sickness, whereas single rotation did not [7, 9]. Rats in the third group were placed in the applicator, but not rotated, while those in the fourth group were neither restrained nor rotated.

Animals were decapitated after rotation or restraint, and their brains were quickly removed. The pons-medulla oblongata was separated by the method of Glowinski and Iversen [3], and stored at —80 °C for assay. Noradrenaline and its major metabolite, MHPG, in samples were extracted and assayed simultaneously by HPLC with an electrochemical detector [2]. Since most of the MHPG in rat brain is present as its sulfate conjugate, total MHPG was measured after its hydrolysis with sulfatase.

The statistical significance of differences was evaluated by Student's t-test.

Results and Discussion

Figure 1 shows the levels of noradrenaline and total MHPG in the brain stem of rats after rotation or restraint for 60 min. The noradrenaline content was not changed after restraint in the applicator for 60 min, and it was slightly, but significantly, decreased after single rotation or double rotation for 60 min. The level of total MHPG in the brain stem was increased markedly and significantly after rotational stimuli, but not simply by restraint. Both single and double rotation increased the level of total MPHG to about 60% more than the control level. These findings demonstrated that both single rotation and double rotation increased the turnover of noradren-aline, suggesting that rotational stimulation activated the noradrenergic neuron system in the brain stem. But, since double rotation induced motion sickness whereas single rotation did not [7, 9], the increased noradrenergic neural activity did not appear to be related directly with the development of motion sickness.

Clinical pharmacological studies have led to a hypothesis for explaining the mechanism of anti-motion sickness drugs. The fact that amphetamine, which releases noradrenaline, is effective in preventing motion sickness suggests that noradrenaline inhibits motion sickness. The anatomical locus of this inhibitory effect of noradrenaline on motion sickness is unknown, but has been suggested to be the noradrenergic neuron system in the vestibular nuclei and the reticular formation in the brain stem [10, 11]. Histochemical studies indicated that the central noradrenergic neuron system originates from the locus ceruleus and the lateral tegmentum, and that from these regions the nerve fibers spread to all regions of the brain, including the brain stem [6]. However, the vestibular nuclei are devoid of noradrenergic termi-nals and the brain stem reticular formation contains only a few fibers [6]. Electrophysiologically, conditioning stimulation of the locus ceruleus has no effect on the neural activity in the lateral vestibular nucleus [1]. Neurons in the medial vestibular nucleus were inhibited by iontophoretic application of noradrenaline, but the effect was not blocked by α- or β-antagonists [4]. The present neurochemical study demonstrated that noradrenergic neuro-transmission in the brain stem was elevated by rotational stimulation, but that the elevation was not specific to motion sickness.

We conclude from this work that the noradrenergic neuron system in the brain stem is not important in development of motion sickness. If the noradrenergic neuron system is involved in motion sickness, the locus for its effect must be in a higher region of the central nervous system, including the arousal-attention system.

References

1   Chikamori, Y.; Sasda, M.; Fujimoto, S.; Takaori, S.; Matsuoka, I.: Locus coeruleus-induced inhibition of the dorsal cochlear nucleus neurons in comparison with the lateral vestibular nucleus neurons. Brain Res. *194:* 53–63 (1980).
2   Firukawa, K.; Karasawa, T.; Kadokawa, T.: An HPLC-ECD analysis of free and conjugated forms of biogenic monoamines and their metabolites in biological samples. Jap. J. Pharmacol. *40:* suppl., p. 149P (1986).

3 Glowinski, J.; Iversen, L.L.: Regional studies of catecholamines in the rat brain. I. J. Neurochem. *13:* 655–699 (1966).
4 Graybiel, A.; Wood, C.D.; Knepton, J.; Parkins, G.F.: Human assay of anti-motion sickness drugs. Aviat. Space Environ. Med. *46:* 1107–1118 (1975).
5 Kirsten, E.B.; Sharman, J.N.: Characteristics and response differences to iontophoretically applied norepinephrine, *d*-amphetamine and acetylcholine on neurons in the medial and vestibular nuclei of the cat. Brain Res. *112:* 77–90 (1976).
6 Moore, R.Y.; Bloom, F.E.: Central catecholamine neuron system: anatomy and physiology of the norepinephrine and epinephrine systems. Annu. Rev. Neurosci. *2:* 113–168 (1979).
7 Morita, M.; Takeda, N.; Kubo, T.; Matsunaga, T.: Pica as an index of motion sickness in rats. ORL (1988).
8 Morita, M.; Takeda, N.; Kubo, T.; Wada, H.; Matsunaga, T.: Effects of anti-motion sickness drugs on motion sickness in rats. ORL (submitted).
9 Takeda, N.; Morita, M.; Kubo, T.; Yamatodani, A.; Wada, H.; Matsunaga, T.: Histaminergic mechanism of motion sickness — neurochemical and neuropharmacological studies in rats. Acta oto-lar. *101:* 416–421 (1986).
10 Wood, C.D.; Graybiel, A.: A theory of motion sickness based on the pharmacological reaction. Clin. Pharmacol. Ther. *11:* 621–629 (1970).
11 Wood, C.D.: Antimotion sickness and antiemetic drugs. Drugs *17:* 417–479 (1979).

Noriaki Takeda, MD, Department of Otolaryngology, Osaka University
School of Medicine, 1-1-50 Fukushima, Fukushima-ku, Osaka 553 (Japan)

Adv. Oto-Rhino-Laryng., vol. 42, pp. 238–241 (Karger, Basel 1988)

Effects of Deuterium Oxide and Ethyl Alcohol on Vestibulo-Ocular Reflex in Rabbits

I. Koizuka[a], *N. Takeda*[a], *T. Kubo*[b], *T. Matsunaga*[a]

[a]Department of Otolaryngology, Osaka University School of Medicine, Osaka;
[b]Department of Otolaryngology, Kagawa Medical College, Kagawa, Japan

Introduction

Ingestion of deuterium oxide or ethyl alcohol induces positional nystagmus. The positional nystagmus is thought to originate in the vestibular end-organs, especially in the semicircular canals, because the positional nystagmus is not observed after labyrinthectomy or plugging of the semicircular canals [1–3]. The dynamic mechanism of the positional nystagmus, however, has not yet been defined.

Based on the torsion pendulum model of the cupula-endolymph system, the relation between angular acceleration and the resulting displacement of the cupula is theoretically a second-order system, which is mainly characterized by long time constant [4, 5].

In the present study, we used the long time constant as an index of the dynamics of the cupula-endolymph system and investigated the effect of deuterium oxide and ethyl alcohol on the cupula-endolymph system in rabbits.

Materials and Methods

Twenty-seven adult, pigmented rabbits, weighing from 3 to 4 kg, were used. Horizontal eye movements were recorded in the dark by means of ENG techniques. Silver needle electrodes were placed at the outer canthi of the rabbits. For measuring the gain of vestibulo-ocular reflex (VOR), experimental animals were placed with their heads on the center of the rotatory table, which was driven by a computer-controlled direct drive motor. They were rotated sinusoidally at the frequencies of 0.033, 0.067, 0.125, 0.25, 0.5 and 1 Hz. The maximum angular velocity of the rotation ranged from 7.9 to 12.6 °/s.

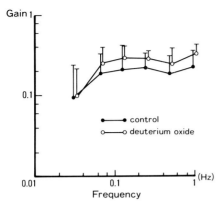

Fig. 1. Gain frequency bode plot of VOR after 30 min of deuterium oxide injection at a dose of 4 ml/kg intravenously in 5 rabbits and that in controls. Closed circles represent the gain of controls and open circles represent that of deuterium oxide. The gains at all frequencies tend to increase compared with the controls. The long time constant in the deuterium oxide treated animals tends to prolong to 2.2 s, whereas the value of controls is 2.0 s.

Gain of VOR was determined as the ratio of slow phase eye velocity relative to the head velocity, and the long time constant of the cupula-endolymph system was then calculated.

Deuterium oxide (purity 99.85%; specific gravity 1.10) and ethyl alcohol (purity 99.5%; specific gravity 0.793) were injected intravenously into rabbits. Control animals were rotated without administration of these substances. The statistical significance of differences was evaluated by the Student's t-test.

Results and Discussion

The gains of VOR at all frequencies tended to increase over the controls 30 min after the administration of deuterium oxide at a dose of 4 ml/kg (fig. 1). Then, the long time constant of VOR was estimated from the gain frequency board plots. The long time constant in the deuterium oxide treated animals tended to prolong to 2.2 s, whereas the value of controls was 2.0 s.

Figure 2 shows gain frequency bode plots of VOR 30 min after ethyl alcohol administration at a dose of 2 ml/kg, and that of the controls. The gains of VOR at all frequencies decreased significantly, in comparison with those of controls. Thus, the long time constant tended to reduce to 1.5 s.

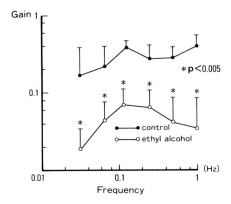

Fig. 2. Gain frequency bode plot of VOR after 30 min of ethyl alcohol injection at a dose of 2 ml/kg intravenously in 6 rabbits and that in controls. Closed circles represent the gain of controls and open circles represent that of ethyl alcohol. Statistically the two groups are significantly different (p <0.005). The long time constant tends to reduce to 1.5 s.

These findings demonstrated that deuterium oxide enhanced the VOR and prolonged the long time constant of VOR and conversely ethyl alcohol decreased the gains of VOR. Since the long time constant mainly represents the dynamics of the cupula-endolymph system, it can be assumed that deuterium oxide and ethyl alcohol affected the cupula-endolymph system in the vestibular end-organs, although some influence of alcohol on the central vestibular system could not be neglected.

The long time constant is dependent upon several factors, such as density of the cupula and the endolymph, viscosity of the endolymph, radius of the semicircular canal, pressure of the endolymph and so on. When some substance was injected intravenously, it is thought to infiltrate to the cupula of the semicircular canal more rapidly than in the endolymph, because it reached the cupula via the capillaries, however it reached the endolymph via another route such as permeation from the stria vascularis. Accordingly, it diffuses more extensively from the blood into the cupula than in the endolymph [6, 7]. When ethyl alcohol whose specific gravity is 0.793 was injected, difference of ethyl alcohol concentration between the cupula and the endolymph occurred. Consequently, the cupula becomes lighter than the endolymph, and then the long time constant of VOR seemed to reduce. It is likely that positional alcohol nystagmus of positive geotropic type was induced by buoyancy resulted from different distributions of ethyl alcohol between the cupula and the endolymph. The hypothesis was supported by the result of deuterium oxide experiment. Deuterium oxide whose specific gravity is 1.10 had the opposite effect on the long time constant of VOR and induced nystagmus of the opposite direction, in comparison with the case of ethyl alchohol. It is probable that since the cupula with deuterium oxide became heavier than the endolymph, the long time constant was prolonged and positional nystagmus of negative geotropic type was induced. Therefore, we concluded that deuterium oxide and ethyl alcohol affect the long time constant by changing the density of the cupula. And positional nystagmus was induced by the bending of the cupula respond to the gravity.

References

1   Kleyn, A. de; Versteegh, C.: Experimentelle Untersuchungen über den sogenannten Lagenystagmus während akuter Alkoholvergiftung beim Kanichen. Acta oto-lar. *14:* 356–377 (1930).

2   Aschan, G.; Bergstedt, M.; Stahle, J.: Nystagmography: toxic states. Acta oto-lar., suppl. 129, pp. 54–58 (1956).

3   Money, K.E.; Myles, W.S.: Heavy water nystagmus and effects of alcohol. Nature, Lond. *247:* 404–405 (1974).

4   Steinhausen, W.: Über die Beobachtung der Cupula in den Bogengangsampullen des Labyrinths des lebenden Hechts. Pflügers Arch. ges. Physiol. *232:* 500–512 (1933).

5   Robinson, D.A.: The use of control system analysis in the neurophysiology of eye movements. Annu. Rev. Neurosci. *4:* 463–503 (1981).

6   Money, K.E.; Johnson, W.H.; Corlett, B.M.A.: Role of semicircular canals in positional alcohol nystagmus. Am. J. Physiol. *208:* 1065–1070 (1965).

7   Reinis, S.; Landort, J.P.; Ewiss, D.S.; Money, K.E.: Effects of deuterium oxide and galvanic vestibular stimulation on visual cortical cell function. J. Neurophysiol. *51:* 481–499 (1984).

Dr. Izumi Koizuka, Department of Otolaryngology, Osaka University School of Medicine, 1-1-50 Fukushima, Fukushima-ku, Osaka 553 (Japan)

Adv. Oto-Rhino Laryng., vol. 42, pp. 242–245 (Karger, Basel 1988)

Modulation of Coordinated Head-Eye Movements by Alcohol and Benzodiazepines

U. Reker, J. Müller-Deile, S. Ehrlich

Universitäts-HNO-Klinik Kiel, Kiel, FRG

Alcohol and hypnotics are known to cause some state of dizziness. We examined isolated eye movements and coordinated head-eye movements to obtain objective information, if this is vestibularly or otherwise induced.

Method

The subjects had to look at one of two light-emitting diodes — subtending an angle of 80° — which were lighted up in an unpredicted time sequence. DC registration of eye movements was effected by the electronystagmographic principle with bitemporal skin electrodes. Recording of head movements was done using a special head-holding device connected to a potentiometer. The velocity of the whole coordinated head-eye movement (i.e. gaze) was obtained by summation of head and eye signals by the computer.

In our *first* study 25 healthy subjects received 2 mg of Flunitrazepam in the evening. Before this and the next morning, the parameters of isolated eye movements and coordinated head-eye movements were measured.

Results (1)

The maximum *velocity* of the isolated eye movement decreased from 417 to 374 °/s. This was significant on the 1% level with the Wilcoxon matched pairs signed rank test. The maximum velocity of the coordinated head-eye movement decreased from 396 to 326 °/s. The additional intake of alcohol (0.5 g/kg) produced a further significant reduction of eye velocity by 25 °/s.

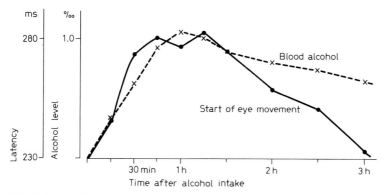

Fig. 1. Curve of blood alcohol level and temporal course of latency prolongation with isolated eye movements.

A *second* study was carried out to analyze the effect of alcohol and its temporal course in more detail. Eighteen healthy subjects drank 0.8 g alcohol/kg and the temporal course of blood alcohol level and performance data were analyzed at intervals of 15 or 30 min up to 3 h. The mean maximum blood alcohol level was 1.07‰ 1 h after intake. After 3 h the alcohol level was still at 0.66‰.

Results (2)

Mean *latency* of *isolated* eye movements before the intake of alcohol was 230 ms. The latency was highly significantly ($p < 0.001$) prolonged to 280 ms 1 h after alcohol intake, but rapidly returned to normal, reaching its original value after 3 h, despite the still high blood alcohol level of 0.66‰ (fig. 1).

This might be explained by some compensatory action or adaptation of the brain, as is known for subjective and psychic effects that are considerably less pronounced in the elimination phase than in the resorption phase despite equal blood alcohol level. The latency data for the *coordinated* head-eye movement showed a very similar temporal course.

The *velocity* of the *isolated* eye movement showed a very different temporal pattern. It decreased from 441 °/s before intake of alcohol to 366 °/s after 1 h, highly significant ($p < 0.001$) with the Wilcoxon matched pairs signed rank test and correlating in temporal course exactly with the blood alcohol level (fig. 2). Three hours after alcohol intake, the eye velocity was

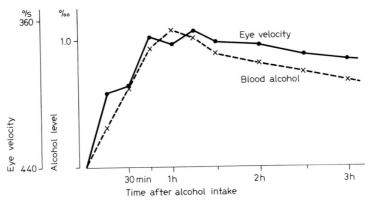

Fig. 2. Curve of blood alcohol level and curve of reduction of eye velocity with isolated eye movements.

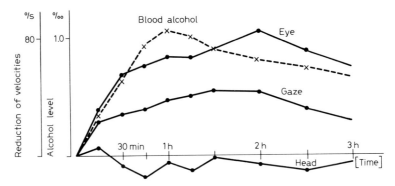

Fig. 3. Coordinated head-eye movement curve of blood alcohol level and temporal course of reduction of eye, gaze and head velocity.

still considerably reduced to 380 °/s. Thus, the reduction of eye velocity correlates exactly with the toxic effect of alcohol. An explanation for this might be that with saccades the eye muscles always have maximum innervation and thus no compensatory reserves.

With the *coordinated head-eye* movement, data were similar (fig. 3). Despite the pronounced reduction of eye velocity, the head velocity was not at all reduced, but slightly higher. This corresponds with the experience that with alcohol levels of 1‰, an effect on skeletal muscle cannot be measured.

The *vestibulo-ocular reflex* as part of the coordinated head-eye movement was not measurably influenced. During the coordinated head-eye movement, the eye reaches its target while the head is still moving (at 190 °/s). From this point of time on, the eye axis in space is vestibularly stabilized. As in our experiments there was no such destabilization of gaze target despite the slightly elevated head velocity, there is no disturbance of the simple vestibulo-ocular reflex.

Thus, the dizziness by benzodiazepines or alcohol with head-eye movement is not caused by a modulation of the vestibulo-ocular reflex, but is particularly due to a reduction of eye velocity.

Priv.-Doz. Dr. med. Ulrich Reker, Universitäts-HNO-Klinik,
Arnold-Heller-Strasse 14, D-2300 Kiel (FRG)

Adv. Oto-Rhino Laryng., vol. 42, pp. 246–249 (Karger, Basel 1988)

Early Symptoms of Side Effects due to Aminoglycoside Antibiotics

Toyoji Miyoshi

ENT Department, Minamikyotobyoin National Sanatorium,
Johyo-shi, Kyoto, Japan

Recently many new aminoglycoside antibiotics have been developed and brought to clinical usage. Aminoglycoside antibiotics have ototoxicity in general. Almost all the new types of them have a tendency to disturb the vestibular function much more than the cochlear function. Also, with the replacement of dehydro streptomycin by sulfate type, the vestibular dysfunction becomes much more frequent than the hearing disturbances as the side effects of aminoglycoside antibiotics. Because of the slow and bilateral progress of vestibular disturbance due to systemic administration of drugs, the subjective symptoms of side effects such as vertigo, do not become evident until the defect has become severe. Therefore, it is very important to detect the vestibular dysfunction in the early stage in cases who are treated with aminoglycoside antibiotics. The diagnostic methods which serve for early detection of bilateral vestibular dysfunction must be established. For this purpose, a questionnaire and a case card were sent to the sanatoriums and hospitals which had a clinic for tuberculosis or urologic diseases. The questionnaire was composed of age and sex of the patient, name and dosage of drugs, kinds and degree of side effects, early symptoms, methods and effect of treatment and others.

Results

The total number of cases who suffered from side effects of aminoglycoside antibiotics was 216 (146 males and 70 females). Their age ranged from 3 to 83 years old. These cases were composed of 198 pulmonary tuberculosis, 5 meningitis, 5 urologic diseases, 4 pneumonia and 4 other diseases. One hundred and eighty-two cases out of 216 were treated with streptomycin sulfate, 2 cases with streptomycin and kanamycin, one with streptomycin, gentamycin and amikacin, 19 cases with kanamycin, 7 with gentamycin, 2 with sisomycin and one each with divecacin, amikacin and micronomycin. The most frequent chief complaint due to the side effects was tinnitus, 107 cases out of 216. The tinnitus was, however, transient in most cases and disappeared within several weeks. Hearing disturbances occurred in 33 cases; however, most of them were not confirmed by means of audiometry. Some cases were without the audiogram before administration, and in the other cases who complained of hearing disturbance the audiograms were unchanged before and after administration. The most frequent vestibular symptom was unsteadiness of gait, seen in 69 cases. They never recognized the ataxic sensation when they kept their heads and bodies stationary. When they moved, however, they felt the unsteady sensation. The cases who complained of dizziness were 28, more than the cases with vertigo. Twenty-two cases complained of vertigo. The reason why the vertigo was not so frequent might be that the vestibular function was disturbed slowly and bilaterally at the same time and by the same degree owing to systemic administration of antibiotics. Twenty-three cases suffered from disequilibrium. Nineteen cases complained of the 'jumbling' phenomenon, not as frequent as was expected. Eight cases complained of paresthesia around the mouth or other parts of the face. Three cases had eruption and 3 other cases had fever.

Among these 216 cases, those who suffered from bilateral vestibular dysfunction owing to aminoglycoside antibiotics were picked up and summarized. Their total number was 97. Seventy-eight cases were treated with streptomycin sulfate, 7 cases with kanamycin, 7 cases with gentamycin, and 5 cases were treated with other aminoglycoside antibiotics. There were several early symptoms of side effects. Some patients complained of more than one as first symptoms. Therefore, the sum of symptoms was much more than the number of cases. The most frequent first symptom was the unsteady sensation of the gait (55 patients) especially in dim illumination. A dizzy sensation was more frequent than vertigo. Seventeen cases recognized a dizzy sensation and 12 cases had vertigo. The complaint of a jumbling sensation induced by the body movement was not as frequent as we expected. Only 10 cases had jumbling phenomena. Close questioning revealed, however, that all our cases had jumbling during the course of illness. Eleven cases complained of tinnitus as a first symptom. Four cases complained of hearing disturbance; however, none of them was certified. The cases who were treated with streptomycin were discussed because the cases who were treated with the other drugs were very few. Their total number was 78. The total doses of streptomycin until the first symptom of side effects was brought about were not uniform. It ranged from 1 to 100 g. In more than half of the cases, the symptom was recognized at a dose of less than 20 g; less than 3 g, 6 cases; 3.1–5 g, 2 cases: 5.1–10 g, 10 cases; 10.1–20 g, 26 cases; 20.1–30 g, 14 cases; 30.1–50 g, 13 cases, and 50.1–100 g, 7 cases. The most important fact was that streptomycin, even at a few doses of less than 5 g could disturb the vestibular function. The duration from beginning of administration to the occurrence of the first symptom was also not uniform. The cases who had their first symptom at less than 5 days were 4; 6–10 days were 9; 11–20 days were 18; 21–30 days were 16; 31–40 days were 8; 41–60 days were 14; 61–100 days were 5; and at more than 101 days were 3 cases. The side effect occurred within one month in more than half of the cases. These facts indicated that we must carefully watch for symptoms, as was mentioned before, especially in the initial 30 days or until doses of the drug reach 20 g.

The complete recovery from side effects of aminoglycoside antibiotics could be seen only in 31 cases. Twenty-eight cases got fairly good compensation and 8 cases got only a slight compensation. Ten cases have not been compensated. The patients who could not achieve complete recovery had many troubles in routine life. Because of the slow and bilateral progress of vestibular disturbance, symptoms were scarcely recognized subjectively until the disturbance had considerably progressed. For the complete recovery from bilateral dysfunction, the early detection of disturbance is essential. The close questioning on the early symptoms, as mentioned above, is important. Besides these, the head shaking reading test is recommended.

The head shaking reading test is composed of two steps. At first, the patient holds some printed matter in front of him. He reads the printed matter whilst his hand is shaking. In the second step, he holds the printed matter tightly in front of him and reads it as his head is shaking. When head shaking is worse than during hand shaking, bilateral vestibular dysfunction is suspected. The relative movement between head and printed matter is the same in these two steps. In the first step the eyes pursue the moving target using the oculomotor system only. In the second step, however, the eyes pursue the target using the oculomotor system and the vestibulo-ocular reflex. The vestibulo-ocular reflex assists the fixation of the eye on the target as the head is moving. In the case of bilateral vestibular dysfunction, the lack of vestibulo-ocular reflex disturbs the eye fixation. The comparison of these two conditions, oculomotor system only and oculomotor and vestibulo-ocular reflex, is very sensitive for the detection of slight bilateral vestibular dysfunction.

T. Miyoshi, MD, 108-I Kamiontani Kuze, Jonyo-shi, Kyoto (Japan)

Adv. Oto-Rhino Laryng., vol. 42, pp. 250–253 (Karger, Basel 1988)

Vestibular Autorotation Testing of Cisplatin Chemotherapy Patients

Geli-Ann Kitsigianis, Dennis P. O'Leary, Linda L. Davis

Department of Otolaryngology-Head and Neck Surgery,
University of Southern California, Los Angeles, Calif., USA

Introduction

Cisplatin is an anti-neoplastic agent which has been shown to be ototoxic [3, 9, 10]. Clinical studies had reported the vestibulotoxic effects as rare [1, 4, 8, 11], relative to the toxic effects on the cochlea. However, we have documented objective changes in the horizontal vestibulo-ocular reflex (VOR) by applying the vestibular autorotation test (VAT) to a group of patients following completion of cisplatin chemotherapy [6]. As a follow-up, this is a preliminary report evaluating possible patterns of change in horizontal gain between weekly treatment courses.

The VAT is a new method of computerized vestibular testing based on 18 s of active head and eye movements over linearly increasing frequencies from 0.5 to 6 Hz [2]. Testing the VOR at frequencies greater than 2 Hz permits monitoring of vestibular pathology which may otherwise have gone undetected [6]. The purpose of this study is to analyze week-to-week changes in horizontal gain following each treatment course of cisplatin.

Methods

Nine patients, 5 with testicular carcinoma (TC) and 4 with pulmonary carcinoma (PC) were used, with TC patients receiving six, and PC patients receiving eight cisplatin treatments, respectively. Patient clinical data and selection criteria were described previously [6]. Selection criteria included: (1) negative radiologic evaluation of the brain; (2) no prior or concurrent exposure to ototoxic medication, and (3) availability for initial pretreatment and subsequent repetitive vestibular testing. The VAT was performed prior to initiation of cisplatin chemotherapy and before each subsequent treatment course.

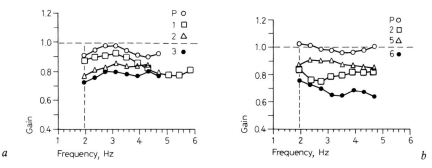

Fig. 1. a Week-to-week changes in horizontal gain versus frequency of one pulmonary carcinoma patient treated with cisplatin. Number of cisplatin treatments: O = pretreatment, □ = 1, △ = 2, ● = 3. *b* Week-to-week changes in horizontal gain versus frequency of one testicular carcinoma patient treated with cisplatin. Number of cisplatin treatments: O = pretreatment, □ = 2, △ = 5, ● = 6.

Methods of data acquisition and analysis were described previously [6], and are summarized in a companion paper [7]. The VAT is a computerized test of 18 s duration, which employs active head movements as high frequency stimuli (0.5–6 Hz) for analyzing the VOR. Eye movements are recorded by electro-oculography. The patient is instructed to fixate on a stationary target while moving the head from side to side in synchrony with audible clicks, which linearly increase in frequency from 0.5 to 6 Hz. Computed VOR parameters are gain and phase, relative to head velocity.

We statistically tested the hypothesis that a decrease in HG which followed completion of cisplatin chemotherapy [6] varied between weekly treatment courses. At the four frequencies, 2.0, 3.1, 3.9, and 5.1 Hz, post-treatment gain values were subtracted from pretreatment values, and the sign of the result was tabulated for the 9 patients following each treatment course. The signs of the 9 values were tested statistically with the distribution-free sign test as a 'paired replicates analysis' [5].

Results

The basis for this study was a significant decrease in horizontal gain and horizontal phase in all 9 patients following completion of 6 cycles of cisplatin chemotherapy [6]. Horizontal gain decreased significantly at 3.1, 3.9 and 5.1 Hz ($p < 0.016$). Horizontal phase decreased significantly at 3.1 and 3.9 Hz ($p < 0.02$). Neither horizontal gain nor phase showed statistically significant changes at 2 Hz. Best estimators of gain changes attributable to cisplatin were −0.15 at 3.1 and 3.9 Hz, and −0.10 at 5.1 Hz. Phase change estimators were −5.0° at 3.1 Hz, and −8.4° at 3.9 Hz ($p < 0.04$).

Results of this study are based on pre- and post-treatment gain values obtained following individual treatment courses. Figure 1a illustrates the weekly changes in horizontal gain for a PC patient. A progressive pattern of decrease in horizontal gain is observed following 1, 2 and 3 treatment courses of cisplatin, such that the most marked decrease in horizontal gain occurred following the final cisplatin treatment. This corresponds to a total cumulative dose of 597 mg of cisplatin. Figure 1b illustrates the weekly progression of change in a testicular carcinoma patient's horizontal gain. Pretreatment gain values were 0.9 or greater, whereas post-treatment gain values decreased markedly. This patient's most severe decrease in horizontal gain occurred following the final (6th) cisplatin treatment. This corresponds to a total cumulative dose of 840 mg of cisplatin. Figure 1b shows that gain values following the 3rd and 5th cisplatin treatments were less than initial pretreatment values, although their order was reversed.

Discussion

One patient from the pulmonary carcinoma group and one patient from the testicular carcinoma group were used to illustrate weekly changes in their respective gain values. These weekly gain changes represent a best estimate of a progression which would be expected from these classes of patients. Results from other patients showed variation in their weekly patterns, attributable to week-to-week test variations [7]. Although these variations precluded determination of a monotonic progression of change in all patients, their trend was toward an overall decrease in horizontal gain following completion of cisplatin chemotherapy. Intermittent (1–2 treatment courses) unavailability of patients for testing prevented documenting statistically significant patterns of change within a 95% confidence interval.

In conclusion, the VAT provides an effective method of monitoring for vestibular pathology. The patients in this study were often very weak both from their disease and from the hematologic side effects of their chemotherapy. However, our experience has been one of excellent patient cooperation. There were no complaints of discomfort. The VAT was frequently performed at the bedside for those patients who felt weak. It is unlikely that this population of cancer patients undergoing chemotherapy would have tolerated or cooperated with other methods of vestibular testing, such as electronystagmography or rotating chairs. Therefore, the VAT is of short duration, can be performed portably, and is not uncomfortable for the patient. We feel that these are important qualities which provide a unique usefulness for the monitoring of cisplatin-induced vestibulotoxicity with the VAT.

References

1   Black, F.O.; Myers, E.N.; Schramm, V.L.; et al.: Cisplatin vestibular toxicity: preliminary report. Laryngoscope *92:* 1363–1368 (1982).
2   Fineberg, R.; O'Leary, D.P.; Davis, L.L.: Use of active head movement for computerized vestibular testing. Arch. Otolaryngol. Head Neck Surg. *113:* 1063–1065 (1987).
3   Higby, D.J.; Wallace, H.J.; Holland, J.F.: Cisplatin: a phase I study. Cancer Chemother. Rep. *57:* 459–463 (1973).
4   Hartwig, S.; Pettersson, U.; Stahle, J.: Cis-diaminedichloro-platinum: a cytostatic with an ototoxic effect. ORL *45:* 257–261 (1983).
5   Hollander, M.; Wolfe, D.A.: Nonparametric statistical methods, pp. 39–50 (Wiley & Sons, New York 1973).
6   Kitsigianis, G.A.; O'Leary, D.P.; Davis, L.L.: Active head movement analysis of cisplatin-induced vestibulotoxicity. Otolaryngol. Head Neck Surg. *98:* 82–87 (1988).
7   O'Leary, D.P.; Davis, L.L.; Kitsigianis, G.A.: Analysis of the vestibulo-ocular reflex using sweep-frequency active head movements. Adv. Oto-Rhino-Laryng. *41:* 179–183 (Karger, Basel 1988).
8   Schaefer, S.D.; Post, J.D.; Close, L.G.; Wright, C.G.: Ototoxicity of low- and moderate-dose cisplatin. Cancer *56:* 1934–1939 (1985).
9   Schaefer, S.D.; Wright, C.G.; Post, J.D.; Frenkel, E.P.: Cisplatinum vestibular toxicity. Cancer *47:* 857–859 (1981).
10 Talley, R.W.; O'Bryan, R.M.; Gutterman, J.U.; et al.: Clinical evaluation of toxic effects of cisplatin-phase I study. Cancer Chemother. Rep. *57:* 465–471 (1973).
11 Wright, C.G.; Schaefer, S.D.: Inner ear histopathology in patients treated with cisplatinum. Laryngoscope *92:* 1408–1413 (1982).

Dennis P. O'Leary, PhD, University of Southern California,
Department of Otolaryngology-Head and Neck Surgery, Vestibular Laboratory,
1420 San Pablo Street Rm C-103, Los Angeles, CA 90033 (USA)

Adv. Oto-Rhino Laryng., vol. 42, pp. 254–259 (Karger, Basel 1988)

The Effects of Baclofen on Periodic Alternating Nystagmus and Experimentally Induced Nystagmus

Takuya Uemura, Hiroaki Inoue, Tetsuo Hirano

Department of Otolaryngology, Faculty of Medicine, Kyushu University, Fukuoka, Japan

Introduction

The role for cerebellar lesions in production of the acquired type of periodic alternating nystagmus (PAN) has been suggested by the findings in clinical and pathological studies. However, the pathophysiology has not been firmly established. Of interest was the fact that two monkeys had PAN appearing only in darkness after removal of the nodulus and ventral uvula [4]. The PAN was abolished in both monkeys by administering baclofen. As the similar type of PAN was found in a patient, we have examined the effects of baclofen on PAN and experimentally induced nystagmus and now report a one-year follow-up study.

Subject

A 64-year-old woman presented with a year's history of increasing oscillopsia mainly in the horizontal plane and sometimes in the vertical or diagonal plane. She first noticed that the environment was moving from the right to the left. The duration was approximately 5 min and at that time she could not remain standing. No cochlear symptom was experienced. Since then similar attacks occurred once or twice a day, mostly at night.

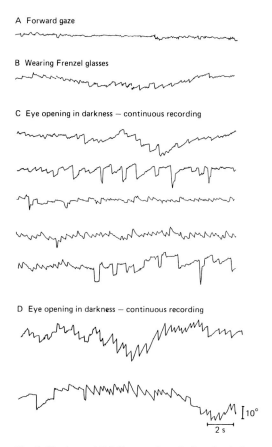

A Forward gaze

B Wearing Frenzel glasses

C Eye opening in darkness — continuous recording

D Eye opening in darkness — continuous recording

10°

2 s

Fig. 1. Horizontal EOG recordings before baclofen treatment.

Methods and Results

The patient's visual acuity was hand motion only in the right eye and 0.1 in the left eye secondary to bilateral cataracts and diabetic retinopathy. The hearing test showed moderate mixed hearing losses in both ears. Standing on both legs with the eyes closed was possible, but standing on one leg with the eyes open was impossible.

No nystagmus was noted in the primary position or on eccentric gaze in either direction (fig. 1a). PAN with variable cycles was observed when wearing Frenzel glasses (fig. 1b) and was recorded by EOG with the eyes

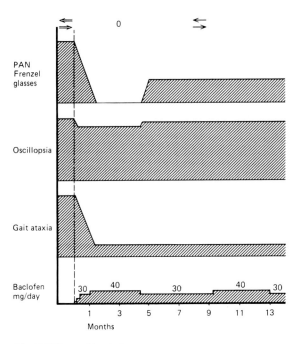

Fig. 2. Effects of baclofen treatment.

closed and open in darkness. A cycle length, for example, was 96 s with a left beating phase of 45 s, a right beating phase of 40 s and two null periods of 5 and 6 s (fig. 1c). Another cycle length was 43 s with a left beating phase of 22 s, a right beating phase of 12 s and two null periods of 4 and 5 s (fig. 1d). The maximum velocity of the slow phase was 40 °/s. No changes in the features of PAN were seen in postural changes. The directions of oscillopsia were similar to those of the quick phase of PAN. Examination of optokinetic nystagmus (OKN) was within normal range, and visual pursuit was slightly hypometric with catch-up saccades. No ocular dysmetria or rebound nystagmus was noted. Caloric tests were active and the rate of visual suppression was 76%, being judged as normal. No other neurological findings were noted. No abnormality was shown except slight cortical atrophy by either metrizamide-CT or magnetic resonance imaging (MRI) scan.

As shown in figure 2, baclofen was given in gradually increasing dosages from 5 to 40 mg/day, and thereafter a daily dose of 40 mg was maintained. On the 12th day after baclofen administration the intensity of PAN began to

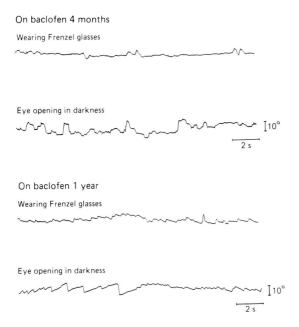

On baclofen 4 months

Wearing Frenzel glasses

Eye opening in darkness

I10°

2 s

On baclofen 1 year

Wearing Frenzel glasses

Eye opening in darkness

I10°

2 s

Fig. 3. Horizontal EOG recordings on baclofen treatment for 4 months and 1 year.

decrease. PAN disappeared under the condition of wearing Frenzel glasses 7 weeks later and under the condition of opening the eyes in darkness 4 months later (fig. 3, on baclofen 4 months). Unsteadiness on walking was markedly improved. The extent of oscillopsia was lessened, but still remained after the disappearance of PAN.

Since she had a transient ischemic attack, baclofen was reduced to 30 mg/day. Thereafter, PAN reappeared under the conditions of wearing Frenzel glasses and opening the eyes in darkness, but to a lesser extent than before baclofen administration (fig. 3, on baclofen one year). Although baclofen was increased to 40 mg/day 2 months later, the intensity of PAN remained unchanged.

No significant differences were found among the examinations of experimentally induced nystagmus and the eye tracking tests which were performed before the treatment, and on the treatment for 4 months and for one year, respectively. Comparison of the test results is shown in table I. No development of side effects was noted during one year's treatment.

Table I. Comparison of test results before and on baclofen treatment

	Before baclofen	On baclofen 4 months	On baclofen 1 year
PAN	+++	–	+
Caloric nystagmus	+	+	+
Visual suppression, %	76	65	80
OKN	near normal	near normal	near normal
OKAN		–	–
Eye tracking	slightly saccadic	slightly saccadic	slighty saccadic

Discussion and Conclusion

Although the efficacy of baclofen on PAN was first reported by Halmagyi et al. [1] and then by others [2, 3], it is not clear whether its beneficial effect lasts while a certain amount of the drug is continued. In our patient complete abolition of PAN had been obtained once, but thereafter only a partial suppression occurred even by its administration for one year. Thus, baclofen does not seem to be a real therapeutic drug for PAN.

Even though it is temporary, the effect of baclofen on PAN would be noteworthy. Baclofen is an analog of the inhibitory neurotransmitter γ-aminobutyric acid (GABA); however, there is no conclusive evidence that actions on GABA systems are involved in production of its clinical effects. In this regard it is of interest that PAN similar to that seen in our patient was found in the monkeys after the nodulus and ventral uvula had been removed, and that the PAN was abolished by baclofen administration [4]. These similarities in the features of PAN have raised suspicion of the existence of nodulus and uvula lesions in our patient. However, neither CT nor MRI scan provided any evidence of lesions in the cerebellum.

The action of baclofen was examined using the examinations of experimentally induced nystagmus and the eye tracking tests on the treatment for 4 months and for one year. No significant differences were found except the effects of abolishing or suppressing PAN when compared with the results before the treatment.

Therefore, the effect of baclofen on PAN in this patient should be ascribed to its action into the neural mechanism other than the direct visual or vestibular pathways.

References

1 Halmagyi, G.M.; Rudge, P.; Gresty, M.A.; Leigh, R.J.; Zee, D.S.: Treatment of periodic alternating nystagmus. Ann. Neurol. *8:* 609–611 (1980).
2 Isago, H.; Tsuboya, R.; Kataura, A.: A case of periodic alternating nystagmus: with a special reference to the efficacy of baclofen treatment. Auris Nasus Larynx *12:* 15–21 (1985).
3 Leigh, R.J.; Robinson, D.A.; Zee, D.S.: A hypothetical explanation for periodic alternating nystagmus: instability in the optokinetic-vestibular system. Ann. N.Y. Acad. Sci. *374:* 619–635 (1981).
4 Waespe, W.; Cohen, B.; Raphan, T.: Dynamic modification of the vestibulo-ocular reflex by the nodulus and uvula. Science *228:* 199–202 (1985).

Takuya Uemura, MD, Department of Otolaryngology, Faculty of Medicine, Kyushu University, Fukuoka 812 (Japan)

Adv. Oto-Rhino Laryng., vol. 42, pp. 260–264 (Karger, Basel 1988)

Effects of Intravenously Given Barbiturate and Diazepam on Eye Motor Performance in Man

Lucyna Schalen[a], Ilmari Pyykkö[b], Kari Korttila[c], Mans Magnusson[a], Hakan Enbom[a]

Departments of Otolaryngology, University Hospitals of [a]Lund, Sweden, [b]Helsinki, Finland, [c]Department of Anesthesiology, University Hospital of Helsinki, Finland

Introduction

Quantification of eye movements is frequently used for estimating the effect of drugs on psychomotor functions. During the last few decades several papers on the effect of oral intake of barbiturates and diazepines on eye movements in man have been published. Unfortunately, due to the pharmacodynamic properties of the drugs, the results from studies after an oral versus intravenous (i.v.) administration are usually not equal. To our knowledge, however, the effects of the drugs following i.v. administration have been the subject of few studies. Nevertheless, knowledge of the effect of i.v. barbiturate and diazepam on eye movements seems motivated because this medication is common in short-term anesthesia, e.g. in outpatients who may return to ordinary daily activities and traffic shortly after the anesthesia. The present report concerns the effects of i.v. given diazepam and barbiturate on voluntary eye movements and vestibulo-ocular reflex, with special regard to their duration.

Material and Methods

Nine paid volunteers, 5 females and 4 males, aged 22–40 years, without previous history of vertigo or neurological disorder, with normal hearing and vision, participated in the study. The test order was randomized according to a latin square design for three separate days with an interval of 2 weeks. The conditions were: control recordings without drugs (C), after i.v. injection of diazepam (D) 0.3 mg/kg body weight and thiopental (B)

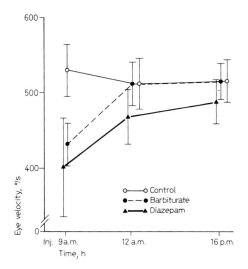

Fig. 1. Velocity of saccade at 60° amplitude at three time points in a day on a control testing and following intravenous injection of diazepam and barbiturate. Mean values and SEM in 9 volunteers are given.

6.0 mg/kg body weight. The drugs were injected at 8 a.m. and the tests were performed at 9 a.m., 12 noon and 16 p.m.

Saccades were tested at 20. 40 and 60° amplitude, pursuit eye movements (PEM) at target velocities of 10–60 °/s and rotation induced nystagmus after a 150 °/s velocity step. Saccadic velocity and latency, velocity of PEM and velocity of slow phase of nystagmus were evaluated on each testing occasion [for details, see Henriksson et al., 1980; Schalen, 1980]. The control results were compared with the results following drugs, using t-test for paired samples and second stage statistics [as in Magnusson, 1986]. The differences were considered significant at $p < 0.05$.

Results

The *velocities of saccades* in the control measurement did not differ at the three different time points of the day. One hour after injection of B as well as D the velocity of saccades was significantly reduced ($p < 0.001$). The reduction was still significant 4 h after D ($p < 0.01$) but not B, however 8 h after injection there were no significant differences between C, B and D,

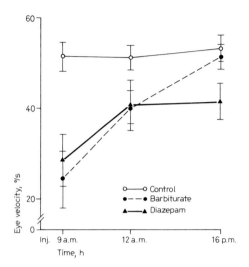

Fig. 2. Velocity of PEM at 60° stimulus velocity at three time points of a day on control testing and following intravenous injection of barbiturate and diazepam. Mean values and SEM in 9 volunteers are given.

respectively (fig. 1). The *latency time* of saccades was a significantly reduced one hour (p <0.05) and 4 h (p <0.01) but not 8 h following B and not at all after D.

The *velocity of PEM* was significantly reduced following administration of both B and D at 1 h (p <0.001) as well as 4 h (p <0.001 B and p <0.01 D). Eight hours after injection of D the velocity of PEM was still significantly reduced (p <0.05) but there was no difference between B and control at this time point (fig. 2). The reduction of PEM velocity was most remarkable at stimulus velocities above the physiological limit of the PEM, i.e. 30 °/s. The maximum *velocity of slow phase of nystagmus* was significantly reduced (t-test p <0.05) 1 h after injection of both B and D, still 4 h after D (p <0.,05) but neither 4 h after B nor 8 h following any of the drugs.

Discussion

The main purpose of the present study was to estimate the duration of the known effects of i.v. medication with diazepam and barbiturate on eye motor performance. According to available data [Tedeschi et al., 1982], the velocity of saccades is not fully normalized 30 min following i.v. injection of diazepam. The present results indicate that the effect on saccade may persist for a minimum of 4 h. Furthermore, an effect on PEM was detectable during at least 8 h.

Differences in pharmacological properties of the two drugs may be sufficient to explain the generally shorter duration of the effect of barbiturate as compared to diazepam. However, biological differences in sensitivity to various drugs and variation in eye motor performance related to individual rhythms of fatigue and vigilance [Schalen et al., 1988] should also be considered, e.g. for recommendations on traffic avoidance following i.v. anesthesia with these drugs.

The sites of action of barbiturates and diazepam in the CNS are not known in detail. It has been speculated that diazepines might primarily affect cerebellar structures [Rottenberger et al., 1981]. However, the results of the present study rather support an assumption that brain stem and supratentorial structures are particularly influenced by the tested drugs. Thus, in our opinion, the marked reduction of velocity of eye movements here demonstrated may reflect a direct action of the drugs on the neuronal populations of the brain stem responsible for execution of proper velocity of eye movements [Keller, 1974; Raphan and Cohen, 1974]. The drugs may also reduce eye motor activity indirectly through a general effect on alertness, exerted either at the brain stem level or supratentorially.

In agreement with Rothenberg and Selkoe [1981], we found no significant effect on saccadic latency following given diazepam whereas reduction occurred following barbiturate. This discrepancy between the two drugs suggests that control of latency time is dependent on structures other than those controlling the velocity of the eye.

In our study reduction of vestibular gain, ascribed to a decrease of the neuronal activity in vestibular nuclei [Prybyla and Wang, 1968], was less pronounced than reduction of velocity of PEM and saccades. However, this parameter may not be sensitive enough to disclose vestibular dysfunction, the time constant being probably more informative [Magnusson, 1986].

Testing of saccades is often proposed for evaluation of psychomotor function [Tedeschi et al., 1982]. The present data suggest that PEM may be more sensitive for this purpose, probably due to an extreme sensitivity of PEM to fatigue and inattention, e.g. when caused by sedative drugs disturbing the continuous velocity adaptation mechanisms.

References

Henriksson, N.G.; Pyykkö, I.; Schalen, L.; Wennmo, T.C.: Velocity patterns of rapid eye movements. Acta oto-lar. *89:* 504–512 (1980).

Keller, E.L.: Participation of medial pontine reticular formation in eye movement generation in monkey. J. Neurophysiol. *37:* 316–332 (1974).

Magnusson, M.: Effect of alertness on the vestibulo-ocular reflex and on the slow rise in optokinetic nystagmus in rabbits. Am. J. Otolaryngol. *7:* 353–359 (1986).

Przybyla, A.C.; Wang, S.C.: Locus of central depressant action of diazepam. J. Pharmac. exp. Ther. *163:* 439–447 (1968).

Raphan, T.; Cohen, B.: Brain stem mechanisms for rapid and slow eye movements. A. Rev. Physiol. *40:* 527–522 (1978).

Rottenberger, S.J.; Selkoe, D.: Specific oculomotor deficit after diazepam. I. Saccadic eye movements. Psychopharmacology *74:* 232–236 (1981).

Schalen, L.: Quantification of tracking eye movements in normal subjects. Acta oto-lar. *90:* 404–413 (1980).

Schalen, L.; Pyykkö, I.; Korttila, K.; Hansson, G.Å.; Magnusson, M.: Velocity of eye movements with special reference to biological rhythm; in Claussen, Computers in neurootology (Elsevier, North-Holland, Amsterdam 1983).

Tedeschi, G.; Smith, A.T.; Sparks, M.G.; Richens, A.: Effect of intravenous diazepam on peak saccadic velocity. Br. J. clin. Pharmacol. *11:* (1982).

Lucyna Schalen, MD, Department of Otolaryngology, University Hospital of Lund, S-221 85 Lund (Sweden)

Adv. Oto-Rhino Laryng., vol. 42, pp. 265–268 (Karger, Basel 1988)

Results of Conservative Treatment of Ménière's Disease and Prediction of the Therapeutic Effect by Hayashi's Quantification Method

Hirofumi Akagi, Takashi Tokita, Hideo Miyata

Department of Otorhinolaryngology, Gifu University School of Medicine, Gifu, Japan

In the treatment of Ménière's disease, the following three subjects were taken into consideration: (1) treatment of vertigo; (2) treatment of damage to the inner ear, and (3) treatment of recurrent attacks of vertigo. The purpose of the present study was to evaluate the effect of conservative treatment of recurrent attacks of vertigo and to predict the effects of the treatment.

Materials and Methods

Fifty-eight patients, diagnosed as having Ménière's disease, were conservatively treated with drug medication. The average interval between spells was between one week and 10 years. All the examinees were diagnosed according to the following criteria specified by Tokita et al. [1975].

History. (1) Recurrent paroxysmal vertigo. (2) Cochlear symptoms associated with vertigo.(3) Unknown causes. (4) No other neurological symptoms; vestibulocochlear symptoms only.

Examination. (1) Perceptive deafness (no sign of retrocochlear deafness). (2) Spontaneous nystagmus and/or CP in caloric response. (3) No other neurological signs; vestibulocochlear signs only.

Twenty-six of the 58 patients were followed up for ten times the average interval between spells, and the following studies were carried out on these 26 patients. (1) The follow-up results were evaluated in accordance with the criteria of the American Academy of Ophthalmology and Otolaryngology [Alford, 1972]. (2) The conditions for the control of spells by the treatment and discrimination between patients showing no definitive spells and those in whom it proved impossible to control definitive spells were studied using Hayashi's [1952] quantification method. In the analysis, control and noncontrol of vertigo were used as outside criteria. As items, length of course, average interval between

Table I. Outside criteria: control and noncontrol of vertigo

Items	Category	Category number	Category	Category number
Length of course	3 months >	1	3 months to 1 year	2
	1–2 years	3	2–5 years	4
	5 years ≤	5		
Average interval	1 month >	1	1–2 months	2
between spells	2 months ≤	3		
Nature of vertigo	rotatory	1	dizziness	2
Severity of vertigo	slight and moderate	1	severe	2
Hearing level	40 dB >	1	40 dB ≤	2
Caloric CP	20% >	1	20–50%	2
	50% ≤	3		

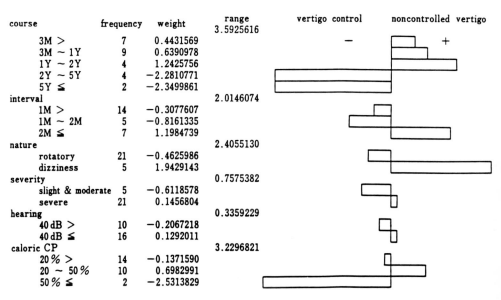

Fig. 1. From left to right, six items, categories, frequencies, weights, ranges and bar graphs of weights.

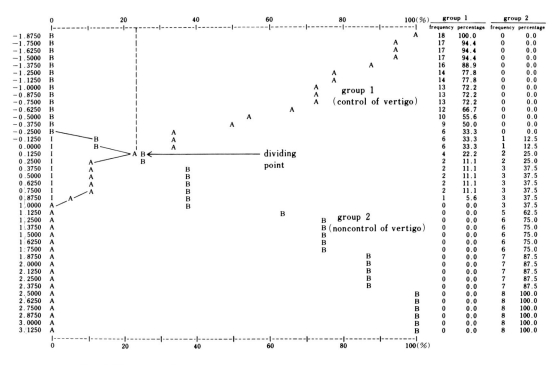

Fig. 2. The cumulative distribution of the sample score.

spells, nature and severity of vertigo, hearing level and caloric CP were used for prediction of the treatment effects. Each item had categories and each category was assigned a number, each of which is shown in table I.

Results

(1) Therapeutic effects were as follows: The 26 patients were divided so that 5 were placed in class A, 12 in class B, 1 in class C and 8 in class D. A total of 18 (69%) in classes A, B and C composed the vertigo-controlled group and 8 in class D the noncontrolled group.

(2) The quantification analysis yielded the following results: The correlation ratio, which indicates the rate at which items explain the outside criteria, was 0.418. The category weight, shown in figure 1, was quantified so that the difference between groups could be made clear. When the category weight

was negative, this indicated a correlation with vertigo control. A positive category weight indicated a correlation with noncontrolled vertigo. The range for an item is the difference between the maximum and minimum values of the category weight. The larger the range, the more significant was the item. The items with the largest ranges were the course and the caloric CP. The sample score, which is the sum of the category weight for each patient, corresponded to the therapeutic effects in 19 of the 26 patients. The partial correlation coefficient indicated a single relation between the outside criteria and each item excluding the influences of other items. The partial correlation coefficients were: length of course, 0.526; nature of vertigo, 0.509; caloric CP, 0.504; average interval between spells, 0.424; severity of vertigo, 0.230; and hearing level, 0.131. The cumulative distribution of the sample score is shown in figure 2. Sample scores are plotted on the ordinate of the graph. The abscissa indicates the percentage cumulative distribution. *A* indicates group 1, i.e. the control group, and *B* indicates group 2, the noncontrol group. The intersection of *A* and *B* is the dividing point. The success rate for this discrimination was 75%.

References

Alford, B.R.: Report of subcommittee on equilibrium and its measurement. Ménière's disease: criteria for diagnosis and evaluation of therapy for reporting. Am Acad. Ophthal. Otolar. *76:* 1462–1464 (1972).

Hayashi, C.: On the prediction of phenomena from qualitative data and the quantification of qualitative data from the mathematico-statistical point of view. Annls Inst. Statist. Mathemat. *3:* 69–98 (1952).

Tokita, T.; Miyata, H.; Hashimoto, M.; Hayano, Y.; Tanaka, K.; Maki, T.; Maeda, M.: Studies on criteria for diagnosis of Ménière's disease and Ménière-like disease. Pract. Otol., Kyoto *68:* 857–866 (1975).

H. Akagi, MD, Department of Otorhinolaryngology, Gifu University
School of Medicine, Gifu 500 (Japan)

Adv. Oto-Rhino Laryng., vol. 42, pp. 269–274 (Karger, Basel 1988)

Intramastoid Drainage Surgery for Ménière's Disease — Critical Analysis of Variation of Surgical Results for Ménière's Disease

Masaaki Kitahara, Kazutomo Kitajima

Department of Otolaryngology, Shiga University of Medical Science, Seta, Otsu, Japan

Introduction

At 8 institutes, our intramastoid drainage surgery — very similar to ours although not identical in each institute [1] — was carried out on 314 cases of Ménière's disease. Our intramastoid drainage surgery consists of the following principles: (1) intramastoid opening of the endolymphatic sac including the rugous portion; (2) the folding back of the lateral wall of the sac, and an insertion of gelfilm into it. The reasonability and safety of our surgery, based on animal examinations and our surgical techniques, were published elsewhere [2, 3]. Results, according to the 1972 AAOO [4] and 1985 AAO-HNS [5] criteria, were reported by each of the surgeons. In this paper, critical analysis of th variations in the results is carried out based on the criteria used and the impressions of the surgeons as expressed in their reports.

Materials

Three hundred and fourteen cases of Ménière's disease underwent intramastoid drainage surgery at the following institutes: 20 cases at Yamagata University by Dr. Koike et al., 63 cases at Tokyo University by Dr. Futaki et al., 36 cases at Shizuoka Hospital by Dr. Matsuoka, 11 cases at Toyama Medical and Pharmacological University by Dr. Mizukoshi et al., 140 cases at Shiga University of Medical Science by Dr. Kitahara et al., 15 cases at Hyogo Medical College by Dr. Kumoi et al., 18 cases at Ehime University by Dr. Yanagihara and 7 cases at Kurume University by Dr. Hirano et al.

Results

Table I shows the results of the intramastoid drainage surgery on 314 cases of Ménière's disease reported by 8 institutes according to the 1972 AAOO and 1985 AAO-HNS criteria for the most part. For example, 1985 AAO-HNS criteria request an assessment of hearing level for four-frequency pure-tone average at 0.5, 1, 2 and 3 kHz. In most institutes in Japan, however, the hearing level for three-frequency pure-tone average, i.e 0.5 kHz + 2 × 1 kHz + 2 kHz/4, are used for assessment, because the hearing level for 3 kHz pure tone is not usually measured in Japan. The other variations from the exact criteria for case selection and/or evaluation of results of each surgeon are shown in table II.

Discussion

Even though the surgical technique is very similar, reported results could differ according to selection of cases, minor changing of criteria for reporting results, etc. Regarding the selection of surgical cases, Matsuoka's cases had been limited to those with a positive glycerol test. This is why his surgical results are considered to be better than those of others. It has been my experience that the results of surgery for cases with a negative glycerol test are worse than those for cases with a positive glycerol test.

All results reported here are based on the 1972 AAOO and 1985 AAO-HNS criteria. Nevertheless, Futaki's report on definitive spells is worse than that of others. This is because he regarded all dizziness as definitive spells. This is a special case. However, it is the general impression of surgeons who analyzed the results that it is difficult to distinguish between definitive spells and others. On the other hand, Kumoi and Hirano's results on definitive spells are much better than others. This is because definitive spells which occurred during the 3-month period following surgery were excluded from their calculations. In most cases, 1–3 months following surgery, vertigo similar to positional vertigo sometimes occurs. After that period, patients are relieved of vertigo. Absence of definitive spells reported by Kumoi and Hirano are 93 and 100%, respectively. If definitive spells occurrinng 3 months following surgery were included in their calculations, their results would be decreased to 47 and 57%, respectively. It seems reasonable to exclude definitive spells occurring at some period of time following surgery from calculation.

Table I. Results of intramastoid drainage surgery for Ménière's disease

Reporter	Koike et al.	Futaki et al.	Matsuoka	Mizukoshi et al.	Kitahara et al.	Kumoi et al.	Yanagihara et al.	Hirano et al.
Number of surgical cases	20	67	36	11	140	15	18	7
Duration between surgery and evaluation, years	2–3	2	1–4	2	2	2	2	0.75–1.75
1972 AAO criteria, %								
Overall level of result								
A	10	27	81	10	13	27	12	14
B	65	21	19	18	58	53	50	86
C	25	3	0	18	7	13	17	0
D	0	49	0	54	22	7	21	0
1985 AAO-HNS criteria, %								
Definitive spells								
Complete		49	100	46	78	93		100
Substantial		45	0	27	16	0		0
Limited		6	0	18	6	0		0
Insignificant		0	0	9	0	0		0
Worse		0	0	0	0	7		0
Hearing Loss								
Improved		42	81	18	15	27		28
Unchanged		39	19	36	70	47		57
Worse		19	0	46	15	26		15

Table II. The variations from the exact criteria for case selection and/or evaluation of results

Futaki et al.	All dizziness is regarded as definitive spells
Matsuoka	Surgical cases are limited to those with positive glycerol test
Kitahara et al.	Definitive spells which occurred during the one-month period following surgery are excluded from calculation
Kumoi, Hirano et al.	Definitive spells which occurred during the 3-month period following surgery are excluded from calculation

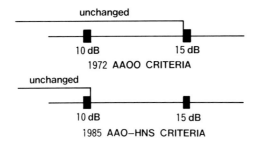

Fig. 1. Difference of area of unchanged hearing between the 1972 AAOO and 1985 AAO-HNS criteria.

Results on hearing loss, according to the 1985 AAO-HNS criteria, e.g. Mizukoshi's, are not good. This might be because the 1985 AAO-HNS criteria regard a minuscule hearing loss or gain, i.e. greater than 10 dB and less than 15 dB on the average of the speech frequencies, as hearing worse or improved, respectively, though this hearing loss or gain is regarded as unchanged in the 1972 AAOO criteria (fig. 1). Actually, it is my impression that the 1972 AAOO criteria for hearing are more practical and more in accordance with the patients' feeling than the 1985 AAO-HNS criteria. There is no description of age in the surgical cases reported. When aged people undergo surgery, the result of hearing cannot simply be compared with that of younger people even if the observation period is 2 years. It should be understood that hearing is influenced by aging, especially in the former cases.

Table III. Reporting according to overall level of result

Class A
1 Absence of definitive spells for described period
2 Hearing improved
Class B
1 Absence of definitive spells for described period
2 Hearing unchanged
Class C
1 Absence of definitive spells for described period
2 Hearing worse
Class D
Failure of control of definitive spells

Table IV. Disability

---

1 No disability
2 Mild disability — intermittent or continuous dizziness/unsteadiness that
  precludes working in a hazardous environment
3 Moderate disability — intermittent or continuous dizziness/unsteadiness that
  results in a sedentary occupation, i.e. desk work
4 Severe disability — symptoms so severe as to exclude gainful employment.

In both the 1972 AAOO and 1985 AAO-HNS criteria, results of definitive spells are treated as more important than those of hearing itself. For example, in the 1972 AAOO criteria, class D is estimated as worse than class C (table III). It should not be permitted to control vertigo at the expense of hearing. In the 1985 AAO-HNS criteria, disability (table IV) due to bilateral deafness — the most unpleasant symptom in advanced cases of Ménière's disease — seems not to be under consideration.

When a selection of surgical cases and/or minor changes in the criteria by each reporter are under consideration, results of our intramastoid drainage surgery could be regarded as very similar, i.e. definitive spells were controlled significantly from 90 to 95%. Hearing was prevented from worsening in 75–85% of cases. However, because of the above-mentioned, it is necessary to increase our efforts to improve criteria for reporting results.

References

1   Kitahara, M.; Takeda, T.; et al.: Experimental and clinical studies on epidural
    drainage surgery. Adv. Oto-Rhino-Laryng., vol. 30, pp. 242–244 (Karger, Basel
    1983).
2   Kitahara, M.; Takeda, T.; et al.: Experimental study on Ménière's disease. Otolaryn-
    gol. Head Neck Surg. *90:* 470–481 (1982).
3   Kitahara, M.; Kitano, H.: Surgical treatment of Ménière's disease. Am. J. Otol.
    *6:*108–109 (1985).
4   Alford, B.R.: Committee on hearing and equilibrium. Am. Acad. Ophthal. Otolaryn-
    gol. *76:* 1462–1465 (1972).
5   Pearson. B.W.; et al.: Committee on hearing and equilibrium guidelines for reporting
    treatment results in Ménière's disease. Otolaryngol. Head Neck Surg. *93:* 579–581
    (1985).

Masaaki Kitahara, MD, Department of Otolaryngology,
Shiga University of Medical Science, Seta, Otsu 520-21 (Japan)

Adv. Oto-Rhino-Laryng., vol. 42, pp. 275–279 (Karger, Basel 1988)

Cochleosacculotomy for Ménière's Disease

Tsun-Sheng Huang, Ching-Chen Lin

Department of Otolaryngology, Chang Gung Medical College, Taipei, Taiwan, ROC

Introduction

The cochleosacculotomy was originally developed by Schuknecht [3] in 1982 on the basis that it enables the creation of a persisting fistula, thus permanently controlling disabling symptoms in patients with Ménière's disease. This hypothesis was at that time supported by animal experiments [4], but contradicted in later studies [2]. Vertigo results achieved have proved comparable to other drainage procedures, although medical literature suggests a greater risk of jeopardising hearing [2, 5].

We analyse herein a series of 29 cochleosacculotomies, emphasising the criteria for selection of candidates relevant to optimum use of this procedure.

Material and Methods

Patient Selection

Other than applying the general principle that surgery for Ménière's disease is only performed where it has proved refractory to medical treatment, our selection of cochleosacculotomy patients was based on the premise that the procedure is designed to relieve vertigo and not to improve hearing. The following criteria for patient selection were therefore employed: (1) intractable vertigo necessitating surgical treatment; (2) poor hearing and a minimal chance of improving it. The latter criterion was primarily assessed by the presence of all or most of the following factors: (1) a non-fluctuating hearing loss; (2) a negative dehydration test; (3) advanced Ménière's disease. In addition, the procedure was employed in cases where an endolymphatic sac shunt was impossible owing to anatomical inaccessibility.

Materials

A total of 29 cochleosacculotomies were performed at Chang Gung Memorial Hospital between May 1984 and August 1986. The male-to-female ratio was 14:15,

Table I. Vertigo results

	N	%
Completely free of vertigo and dizziness	8	28
Adjunctive spells and/or instability	16	55
Recurrent vertigo	5	17

Table II. Hearing results

	N	%
PTA loss above 15 dB	6	21
SDS loss above 15%	9	31
PTA loss at 4 kHz above 15 dB	7	24
PTA loss at 8 kHz above 15 dB	14	48

respectively, with an age range of 24–66, the average being 51. Nineteen patients were aged 50 and over, 9 of whom were 60 or over. Twenty-two cases were on the left ear, and 7 on the right, while the duration of symptoms prior to surgery varied from 1 to 26 years, with an average of 5.2 years. Preoperative pure tone average (PTA) results at 500 Hz, 1, 2 and 3 kHz ranged from 10 to 110 dB, with a mean of 65 dB. Eighteen patients scored a PTA of over 60 dB. Preoperative speech discrimination scores (SDS) ranged from 0 to 100%. All patients had a non-fluctuating hearing loss evidenced by serial audiograms, and a negative dehydration test. The duration of follow-up from surgery to the last examination varied between 7 and 32 months, the average being 17 months.

Since a considerable proportion of those fulfilling the criteria for selection were elderly and candidates for a labyrinthectomy, we have compared cochleosacculotomy results among those patients aged 60 and over, with labyrinthectomy results among patients in the same age range. Twelve out of a total of 54 labyrinthectomised patients were utilised, with a minimum follow-up period of 7 months.

Surgical Technique
Schuknecht's [3] technical details were generally followed, with the exception only that all patients underwent the shunt under general anaesthesia via a postauricular approach exclusively using a 2-mm right-angled hook.

Results

Vertigo results are tabulated in table I and hearing results, as compared with the latest postoperative audiogram, in table II. Results were comparable

Table III. Cochleosacculotomy versus labyrinthectomy results among those of 60 years of age and above

	Cochleosacculotomy		Labyrinthectomy	
	N	%	N	%
Completely free of vertigo	2	22	0	0
Adjunctive spells and/or instability	6	67	10	83
Recurrent vertigo	1	11	2	17

with those of Schuknecht [3, 5], who recently reported a 73% success rate in eliminating definitive vertigo attacks, while a hearing loss of 15 dB or more was recorded among 45% of 90 cases followed up for 22 months.

In our series we encountered 2 patients with chronic otitis media and Ménière's syndrome, who had a dry inactive drum perforation and a sclerotic mastoid. Both patients on whom a tympanoplasty was simultaneously performed were totally relieved of definitive spells, while there was an improvement of hearing and closure of the air-bone gap. Of 2 patients who had experienced a recurrence of vertigo following an endolymphatic mastoid shunt, one resulted in relief of symptoms. We failed to control vertigo in one of 2 patients with bilateral Ménière's disease who had both already undergone a sac shunt on the contralateral ear. Vertigo was relieved and hearing conserved in 2 patients who had vestibular Ménière's disease combined with anatomical anomalies precluding a shunt procedure.

The greatest hearing improvement achieved was from PTA 97 to 75 dB, and from SDS 40 to 80%, a gain arguably attributable to fluctuations in hearing. The worst hearing deterioration meanwhile, was from PTA 45 to 86 dB and SDS 84 to 60%.

Cochleosacculotomy versus labyrinthectomy results among those of 60 years of age and over, as summarised in table III, reveal control of definitive spells to be similar between the two procedures.

Discussion

The cochleosacculotomy was developed by Schuknecht [3, 4] on the basis that the otic-periotic shunt should theoretically prevent distension and ruptures of the endolymphatic system, therefore alleviating vertigo; and that experimental evidence indicated the potential creation of a persisting fistula, between the endolymphatic and perilymphatic spaces, by a needle puncture of the cochlear duct in association with fracture of the osseous spiral lamina.

While animal experiments [2] have since proved contradictory on the issue of the possibility of creating a permanent fistula, clinical data evidences the suppression of vertigo achieved to be comparable to that in other non-destructive surgery for Ménière's disease [1–3, 5], although there is a higher risk to hearing. Furthermore, while Schuknecht [3] himself recognised that there are still problems with the cochleosacculotomy, Thomsen and Bretlau [6] suggested that most conservative therapies for Ménière's disease are non-specific. Indeed, we would speculate that all such procedures may merely induce a temporary remission of the disease process [1].

While the high incidence of a deterioration in hearing following this procedure is a clear drawback, there are numerous advantages in that the technique is simple and easy to perform; there is a low morbidity rate; the procedure can be performed under local anaesthesia (even though we mostly used general in this series); and vertigo results compare favourably with other conservative surgery for Ménière's disease.

The aforementioned advantages and disadvantages of this procedure appear to support the selective use of such for the alleviation of vertigo either where sac surgery is not a viable option, or in advanced cases of Ménière's disease, where hearing is poor and evidence suggests a minimal chance of improving it, i.e. there is a non-fluctuating hearing loss and a negative dehydration test.

Furthermore, as most patients fulfilling such criteria for selection would alternatively be candidates for a labyrinthectomy, we would strongly advise that a cochleosacculotomy be performed before resorting to destructive surgery. Not only do our results show the two procedures to be equally efficacious in vertigo control, even among elderly patients, but a cochleosacculotomy can be performed under local anaesthesia and is less radical in that the inner ear structure is preserved.

Conclusion

Clinical results support the use of a cochleosacculotomy prior to resorting to destructive surgery for the control of intractable vertigo in Ménière's disease, or where sac surgery is not a viable option. Unfortunately, however, the creation of a permanent fistula, the main objective pursued by the medical profession in endolymph drainage operations, appears to remain only a remote possibility.

References

1   Huang, T.S.; Lin, C.C.: Endolymphatic sac surgery for Ménière's disease: a composite study of 339 cases. Laryngoscope *95:* 1082–1086 (1985).
2   Montandon, P.B.; Hausler, R.J.; Kimura, R.S.: Treatment of endolymphatic hydrops with cochleosacculotomy. Otolar. Head Neck Surg. *93:* 615–621 (1985).
3   Schuknecht, H.F.: Cochleosacculotomy for Ménière's disease: theory, technique and results. Laryngoscope *92:* 853–858 (1982).
4   Schuknecht, H.F.: Cochlear endolymphatic shunt. Am. J. Otolaryngol. *5:* 546–548 (1984).
5   Schuknecht, H.F.: Endolymphatic hydrops: Can it be controlled? Ann. Otol. Rhinol. Lar. *95:* 36–39 (1986).
6   Thomsen, J.; Bretlau, P.: General conclusions; in Pfaltz, Controversial aspects of Ménière's disease, pp. 120–136 (Thieme, Stuttgart 1986).

Tsun-Sheng Huang, MD, Department of Otolaryngology,
Chang Gung Memorial Hospital, 199 Tung Hwa North Road, Taipei, Taiwan (ROC)

Adv. Oto-Rhino-Laryng., vol. 42, pp. 280–283 (Karger, Basel 1988)

Indications and Results of Neurovascular Decompression of the Eighth Cranial Nerve for Vertigo, Tinnitus and Hearing Disturbances

H. Ryu[a], *K. Uemura*[a], *T. Yokoyama*[a], *M. Nozue*[b]

Departments of [a]Neurosurgery and [b]ENT, Hamamatsu University School of Medicine, Handa-Cho, Hamamatsu, Japan

It is said that vascular compression against the 8th cranial nerve can cause vertigo, tinnitus and hearing disturbances. However, no one has clearly identified clinical characteristics of the neurovascular compression syndrome of the 8th cranial nerve. Therefore, we analyzed the surgical results of our neurovascular decompression for the 8th cranial nerve.

From December 1982 through April 1987, we performed neurovascular decompression in 27 patients (12 males) with vertigo, tinnitus and/or hearing disturbances (table I). Three patients had vestibular symptoms (vertigo) only, 10 patients had vestibular and cochlear (tinnitus and/or hearing disturbances) symptoms, 10 patients had cochlear symptoms only and 4 patients had cochlear symptoms plus hemifacial spasm. Complete neuro-otological work-ups, auditory brain-stem evoked responses (ABR), air CT and bilateral vertebral angiography were performed preoperatively in all patients. We analyzed each symptom individually. In the 13 patients with vertigo, vascular compression on the 8th nerve was confirmed in 8 patients, who all became symptom-free following neurovascular decompression. Five patients with vertigo had no clear neurovascular compression and vertigo has not changed except for one patient whose symptoms (vertigo and tinnitus) have gradually disappeared in 6 months thereafter (table II). Vertigo due to neurovascular compression was of rotatory or horizontal type and usually had a very short duration (a few seconds to a few minutes). It was always accompanied by tinnitus, sensory-neural hearing disturbance and decreased or absent caloric response on the affected side (table III). On the other hand, the patients who had no neurovascular compression had various kinds of symptoms: 3 patients had positioning vertigo, one had dizziness and one had

Table I. Cases of the 8th cranial nerve dysfunctions

Symptoms	Number	
Vestibular	3	
Vestibular + cochlear	10	} 13
Cochlear	10[1]	
Cochlear + facial spasm	4	} 24
Total	27	

[1] Nerves were cut in 3 cases

Table II. Results of NVD for vertigo

Operative findings	Results		
	no vertigo	unchanged	worse
NVC +	8 (100%)	0	0
NVC −	1	4	0
Total (13)	9 (70%)	4	0

NVD = neurovascular decompression; NVC = neurovascular compression.

Table III. Vertigo due to NVC

Case	Type of vertigo	Duration of vertigo	Caloric response	Tinnitus	Hearing
2	rotatory horizontal	2–3 s	↓	+	↓
7	rotatory	2–3 min	↓	+	↓
8	rotatory	2–3 min	↓	+	↓
10	rotatory	2–3 min	↓	+	↓
13	rotatory	20–30 s	↓	+	↓
17	rotatory	2–3 min	↓	+	↓
19	rotatory	1 min	↓	+	↓
24	rotatory	2–3 h	↓	+	↓

Table IV. Vertigo without NVC

Case	Type of vertigo	Duration of vertigo	Caloric response	Tinnitus	Hearing
1	positioning rotatory headache	few seconds	↓	+	↓
3	positioning rotatory	few seconds	↓	–	normal
6	rotatory dizziness	few min —3 days	↓	+	↓
14	blackout spell	few seconds	↓	+	↓
16	positioning, rotatory	less than 30 s	normal	–	normal

blackout spells. Some even had normal hearing and/or caloric response (table IV). It is our impression that rotatory or horizontal vertigo of very short duration accompanied by tinnitus, decreased hearing and caloric response on one side is very likely due to the neurovascular compression syndrome of the 8th cranial nerve.

As for tinnitus, we confirmed neurovascular compression in 16 cases with tinnitus. One showed marked degeneration of the 8th cranial nerve which was sectioned. Neurovascular decompression was performed in 15 cases, and only 8 have been free from tinnitus postoperatively. It is interesting that, in all patients who had normal hearing preoperatively, neurovascular decompression alleviated the tinnitus (table V). On the other hand, only 4 out of 11 patients who had decreased hearing on the same side preoperatively became free from the tinnitus following the procedure (table VI). We tried to identify the characteristics of the tinnitus due to neurovascular compression. However, some patients had pulsatile tinnitus while others had continuous high-pitched tinnitus, some were accompanied by vertigo, others by hemifacial spasm and still others by hearing disturbance at the same time. There are no special features of tinnitus due to neurovascular compression. However, it is our impression that pulsatile tinnitus alone or tinnitus accompanied by

Table V. Results of NVD for tinnitus with normal hearing

Operative findings	Results		
	no tinnitus	unchanged	worse
NVC +	4 (100%)	0	0
NVC −	0	2	0
Total (6)	4 (67%)	2	0

Table VI. Results of NVD for tinnitus with decreased hearing

Operative findings	Results		
	no tinnitus	unchanged	worse
NVC +	4 (36%)	$7 + 1^1$	0
NVC —	$1 + 2^1$	3	0
Total (18)	7 (39%)	11	0

[1] Nerves were cut.

hemifacial spasm or vertigo of short duration is very likely due to neurovascular compression syndrome, and that such cases should be explored before hearing disturbance develops.

Eighteen patients had sensorineural hearing disturbances and 11 had neurovascular compressions. One showed marked degeneration of the 8th cranial nerve which was cut. We performed neurovascular decompression in the other 10 patients, but no one's hearing was recovered. The results led us to the conclusion that decreased hearing is not the indication of neurovascular decompression.

Air CT is sometimes helpful to detect compressing vessels, especially when the vessels compress the 8th cranial nerve around the internal auditory canal. ABR, on the other hand, is not useful for the diagnosis of neurovascular compression syndrome of the 8th cranial nerve.

H. Ryu, MD, Department of Neurosurgery, Hamamatsu University School of Medicine, 3600 Handa-Cho, Hamamatsu 431-31 (Japan)

Adv. Oto-Rhino-Laryng., vol. 42, pp. 284–286 (Karger, Basel 1988)

Long-Term Relief by Caloric Stimulation in the Treatment of Vertigo

Y. Umeda, M. Nakajima

ENT Department, Kanto Central Hospital, Kamiyohga, Setagayaku, Tokyo, Japan

We have been searching for an effective therapy for attacks of vertigo with nystagmus, especially attacks of long duration, more than 5 days, for example vestibular neuronitis or sudden deafness with vertigo. Generally, in the acute stage of vertigo, tranquilizers and antiemetics are prescribed. However, we do not like to use these drugs from morning till night for more than 5 days. Pursuing another approach, we also know that severe nystagmus can be blocked by caloric nystagmus.

A spontaneous, leftward, horizontal nystagmus caused by right inner ear disorder, for example, can be stopped by pouring cold water into the left ear. This method, however, only brings relief for 3 min or less. Thus, in our experimentation, we concentrated on finding a way to prolong this caloric stimulation, so that relief could last far longer with neither caloric nystagmus nor spontaneous nystagmus reappearing.

Method

In our testing, we achieved success by dripping cold water onto the external auditory canal. Our procedure was as follows: (1) a 500-ml plastic bottle for drip infusion is used; (2) cold water of 20 °C (68 °F) is poured in through a cut in the side of the bottle; (3) this water is then dripped into the ear; (4) the terminal of the infusion line ends over the external auditory canal of the supine patient; (5) a bowl to catch the water spill is placed below the ear; (6) the drip speed is regulated by a clip; and (7) before the bottle empties, more cold water is added.

With the aid of this method, we administered caloric stimulation to the patients, every day for 10 h during the period of 5 days. Perhaps the reader may be surprised at this method of treatment which applies caloric stimulation of 10 h duration and, what is more, for a period of 5 days. The reader may well have the following questions: For example, the first is whether caloric stimulation of long duration might have some bad influences on the inner ear. At the present stage we cannot solve this problem. But our patients have neither vertigo nor deafness • tinnitus during 10 months since their treatment. We would like to stress that the patients are in good condition at present.

The second question is whether caloric nystagmus really continues for more than 10 h. The answer is in the affirmative, for the following reason: after the 10-hour administration of caloric stimulation, we stopped the cold water drip. Spontaneous nystagmus then reappeared.

Following animal experiments, it is believed that caloric nystagmus did not last long. However, in our clinical experience, caloric nystagmus continued for 10 h. This is based on fact.

The third question is whether there is no response decline phenomenon. We cannot yet clarify whether the slow phase velocity of caloric nystagmus is weakened or not. In our experience, however, even on the fifth day, we could evoke caloric nystagmus with the same method applying cold water at the same temperature.

Case Presentation

Case 1
This is a typical case. A 60-year-old female with vertigo was hospitalized at the end of September 1986. Before admission she felt dizzy for three days and had such severe nausea that she could neither walk nor eat. The patient was lying supine with her eyes firmly closed. When she was forced to open her eyes, leftward spontaneous nystagmus was noticed. We diagnosed her disease as disorder of the right inner ear. The patient was given the caloric stimulation in the left ear. Forty seconds after commencing pouring of the cold water, no spontaneous nystagmus was detected. The patient reported that the dizziness had ceased. Some tens of seconds later, there appeared rightward caloric nystagmus which resulted in dizziness in the direction opposite to that experienced before the injection. The clip regulating drip speed was adjusted so that spontaneous and caloric nystagmus could offset each other. Two hours later when caloric stimulation was stopped, the leftward spontaneous nystagmus reappeared; the dizziness was still noticed. Therefore, the injection was given again until 9 o'clock in the evening. For the following 4 days, from morning until bedtime, we conducted a similar procedure, which so far appears to have permanently eliminated vertigo in this patient. On the sixth day after admission we could recognize spontaneous nystagmus, however this patient did not longer feel severe vertigo.

Case 2
In this case we have administered inner ear anesthesia, injecting lidocaine into the middle ear, as a therapy for positional vertigo of benign paroxysmal type. At present, the weak point of this method is that a severe vertigo arises. In order to overcome this undesirable side effect, we tried applying the prolonged caloric stimulation to this vertigo.

Discussion

So far, we have seen that caloric stimulation blocks the vertigo due to inner ear disorder or to inner ear anesthesia.

Some questions now arise. (1) Can the vertigo provoked by caloric stimulation to the right ear be counterbalanced by caloric stimulation to the left ear? (2) Is the vertigo suddenly caused by the disorder in the right ear counterbalanced by the disorder in the left inner ear? (3) Can the bilateral application of inner ear anesthesia prevent the appearance of vertigo?

These possibilities are all denied. When cold water is poured bilaterally, horizontal caloric nystagmus does not appear but upward vertical nystagmus accompanied by vertigo appears. Bilateral inner ear disorders provoke downward vertical nystagmus and vertigo. And bilateral inner ear anesthesia provokes downward vertical nystagmus and vertigo.

It seems that the nystagmus caused by cold water injection into the right canal has not only a leftward component, but also an upward one. In the case of the nystagmus due to the disorder of the right inner ear, both a leftward and a downward component is to be considered. Similarly, the nystagmus caused by inner ear anesthesia on the right has a component not only leftward but also downward. Therefore, we have to be concerned with the counterbalance of horizontal and vertical components in order to block nystagmus.

Conclusion

In conclusion, the vertigo coming from inner ear disorder or inner ear anesthesia can be stopped by caloric stimulation, but counterbalance of other combinations of nystagmus seems to be theoretically impossible.

Y. Umeda, MD, ENT Department, Kanto Central Hospital,
6-25-1 Kamiyohga, 158 Setagayaku, Tokyo (Japan)

Adv. Oto-Rhino-Laryng., vol. 42, pp. 287–289 (Karger, Basel 1988)

Comparative Study of Two Types of Exercise Treatment for Paroxysmal Positioning Vertigo

Marcel E. Norré, A. Beckers

Departments of Otoneurology and Equilibriometry, University Hospitals, University of Leuven, Leuven, Belgium

It has become a generally accepted notion that some types of vertigo can be cured by exercise treatment. However, it has to be emphasized that a well-founded indication is a prerequisite for success. Only 'provoked' vertigo is an indication for such a method of treatment. Provoked vertigo is vertigo elicited by movement or change of position [1]. The causative basic condition is a permanent peripheral vestibular trouble, characterized by a steady state of dysfunction. The goal of exercise treatment is to stimulate readaptation in the central processing in the way that the final goal of balance function is re-achieved. Repeatedly exposing the balance system to the effect of the dysfunction is the very stimulus for developing the required adaptation. It is by eliciting vertigo that the adaptive processes are stimulated.

Vestibular habituation training (VHT) has been developed based upon these premises [1]. Very satisfying results have been obtained. The particular feature of the VHT technique is that the treatment schedule is specific, elaborated and adapted to the needs of each particular patient. The exercises stimulate a progressive development of adaptation by repeating the movements provoking vertigo. VHT can be applied for every kind of provoked vertigo, provided it is of peripheral origin. Patients with typical benign paroxysmal positioning vertigo (BPPV) belong to this category.

For BPPV an alternative exercise scheme has been proposed [2], whereby one single brisk maneuver should reduce the vertigo in one session. This technique is based upon the assumption that the BPPV is caused by cupulolithiasis and the brisk manouevre should dissolve the debris on the cupula of the posterior semicircular canal. The patients selected for rehabilitation treatment were submitted to the VHT test battery, which consists of 19 manoeuvres [1].

Table I. Results by brisk method (group A) and VHT (group B)

	Evaluation No.			Final
	1	2	3	
A. Mean of the scores				
Group A (n = 23)	113	121	14	5
Group B (n = 28)	144	66	43	0
B. Number of positive cases				
Group A (n = 23)	23	11*	5	1
Group B (n = 28)	28	19	8	0

Follow-up evaluations: 1 = onset; 2 = after 1 week; 3 = after 2 weeks. E = End evaluation after 6–8 weeks. *VHT exercises started for the 11 cases (group A2).

For each manoeuvre it was noted whether vertigo was elicited or not, whether the vertigo was described as typically rotatory or as a rather atypical dizziness (A). Intensity (I) and duration (T) of the vertigo were estimated. These items were used for computing a score according to the formula $f(A)g(I)\log10(T)$. The sum of the scores for the positive manoeuvres gave a 'total score', characterizing the situation of the case. The positive manoeuvres are used as specific exercises.

In this study the patients with manoeuvres typically positive were considered, i.e. the patients manifested a typical, i.e. rotatory, vertigo by executing the manoeuvre and a nystagmus (of the transitory type) was observed simultaneously. Only cases with a positive reaction for manoeuvres towards one side ('unilateral' cases) were taken into consideration.

By repeating the evaluation on the VHT test battery during the follow-up and comparing the scores obtained, progression of the therapy was assessed. The patients were re-evaluated after one week. If the score had become zero, an appointment was made for final evaluation 5 weeks later. If the score was still positive, treatment was continued and re-evaluations were done after one week each time until the score had become zero. In each case a final evaluation was done 6 weeks after beginning of treatment.

Fifty-one 'unilateral' cases were treated either with the classical progressive VHT technique (28 cases — group B), or with the brisk technique (23 cases — group A). After one week the patients unchanged by the brisk technique were switched over to a treatment with VHT (group A2 — table I).

Table I shows that in the present comparative study, a higher proportion of the patients treated by the brisk method (12 of 23 = 52.17%) reached a zero score after one week than did the patients treated by VHT (9 of 28 = 32.14%). However, this difference is not statistically significant. Moreover, the patients treated by VHT exercises and being still positive after one week of treatment (n = 19) nevertheless showed a therapeutic effect: the mean of the scores was significantly reduced (144–66), whereas for those treated by the brisk method and still positive after one week, unchanged values (113–121) were observed.

This means that, by the brisk method, a complete result is obtained at once or there is absolutely none as, after one week, half of the cases treated by this method were unchanged. On the contrary, all the cases treated by VHT indicated a progression by a significant reduction of the score. The same proportion of group A2 (5 of 11 = 45.45%) is completely free of vertigo after one week of VHT, as occurred in group B for the first week of treatment. The final result is equal for both groups.

Accordingly, the brisk method appeared to be interesting as it was possible to cure the patient completely in only one session, but this technique is only valuable for 'unilateral' cases and appears to be successful in only 50% of the cases treated. Lack of effect can be overcome by switching over to VHT treatment. The VHT method had the same favourable final result for identical cases in group B. The effect was more progressive. When the application of this brisk technique appears to be difficult as, for example, in aged or obese patients, when there is a painful spinal cord, etc., the same favourable result can finally be obtained by the VHT, the progressive method. The latter keeps its universal applicability. It is the only technique indicated for 'bilateral' and 'atypical' cases with provoked, positioning vertigo. Moreover, it serves as a rescue for the cases where the brisk method has no success.

References

1   Norré, M.E.: Rationale of rehabilitation treatment for vertigo. Am. J. Otolaryngol. *8:* 31–35 (1987).
2   Toupet, M.; Semon, A.: La physiothérapie du vertige paroxystique bénin; in Hausler, Les vertiges d'origine périphérique et centrale, pp. 21–27 (IPSEN, Paris 1985).

Prof. Dr. M. Norré, Schotstraat 2, B-3020 Herent (Belgium)

Adv. Oto-Rhino-Laryng., vol. 42, pp. 290–293 (Karger, Basel 1988)

Curing the BPPV with a Liberatory Maneuver

A. Semont[a], G. Freyss[b], E. Vitte[b]

[a]Vestibular Rehabilitation and [b]ENT Department, Hôpital Lariboisière,
Paris, France

Introduction

From 1897, when Adler first described paroxysmal vertigo, to 1952 with
the well-known 'Hallpike maneuver' [1], then, later, with studies of nystagmus by Katsarkas and Outerbridge [2], Baloh et al. [7], and Stahle and
Terrins [6], benign paroxysmal positional vertigo (BPPV) has been well
known.

Even if there are still discussions about the cause, our preoccupation was
with the treatment. No medical treatment proved to be effective. We know
that attacks spontaneously disappear mostly in 1 month. But recurrence
comes 1 year later after the primary attack and afterwards it may recur
every 3 months and sometimes never disappears. This means that medical
treatment is a psychological security. Surgical treatment was proposed in
1974 by Gacek [3] with good results but with the possibility of hearing loss
after surgery.

In 1979, Norre and Dveerd [4] suggested applying to BPPV patients
what we had already carried out in other patients with vestibular diseases,
since 1968 with the collaboration of Sterkers [8]: vestibular habituation
training. Two hypotheses of what generates BPPV topped all others: (1)
cupulolithiasis, as described by Schuknecht [5]; (2) heavy material floating in
the endolymph, as suggested by Hall, MacClure et al.

In our opinion, these two considerations are complementary, leading to
the same mechanical disturbance of the cupula of the posterior semicircular
canal. In these conditions the density of the cupula is modified and then acts
as an otolithic system under gravity.

One of us (A. Semont) suggested a maneuver that would free the cupula
using the addition of the pressure of the endolymph and the inertia of the

'heavy materials'. The results were so extraordinary and unbelievable that nothing was said except allusions to the facility of curing BPPV [8].

Then Brandt and Daroff suggested a therapy with the idea of habituation training performed by the patient himself. In their published results, one could read that about one third of the patients were cured after one maneuver. That confirmed our astonishing results after only one maneuver.

It is this maneuver, which has been performed on over a thousand patients, that we present here.

Cases and Method

Among the patients treated, only 711 of them have been correctly recorded. Most of these cases were idiopathic and some were post-traumatic. Age range was between 55 and 60 years; 64% of the patients were female. Post-traumatic patients were mainly between 20 and 45 years and the idiopathic patients were from 45 to 85 years old.

No hearing problems were related to BPPV. Caloric tests showed such abnormalities as : slightly reduced or increased values (sick ear). When EOG was done one month after therapy, everything was back to normal (sick ear).

In our opinion the main characteristics of BPPV are: (1) the nystagmus is, when observed on a well-centered eye in orbit, of a rotatory type, rolling toward the lower ear; (2) the nystagmus is inverted when the patient is brought back to the primary position (orthostatism); (3) the provoked nystagmus stops after 30 s maximum, this being correlated with the decrease in the vertigo as felt by the patient.

The Maneuver

The patient is laid on the ipsilateral side to the sick ear with his head slightly declined. The nystagmus can appear: in this condition one must wait until it stops. If nothing happens the head is turned 45° facing up in order to have the cupula in a perpendicular plane to gravity. In this position, after a variable latency, the paroxysmal rotatory nystagmus rolling toward the examination table appears. One waits until it has completely stopped and then the patient is left in this position for 2 or 3 min.

Then, holding patient's head and neck with two hands, he is *swung* quickly to the opposite side. The speed of the head must be zero at the very moment the head touches the examination table. Then a rotatory nystagmus appears *still* rolling toward the sick ear which is now the *higher* one. *It must not be an inverted nystagmus.* The nystagmus is slightly different: wide amplitude, slower frequency, not so paroxysmal as the original one.

If nothing happens the head is slowly turned nearly to 90° facing up and then quickly turned to 45° facing down. Then the nystagmus occurs. The patient must stay in this last position for at least 5 min and is brought back to orthostatism very, very slowly.

The patient is then asked to keep his head absolutely vertical in space during at least 48 h day and night. He is asked to avoid fast head movements upward or downward and not to sleep on the vertigo-generating side for a week. If the maneuver is not successful, it is performed again a week later.

Results

After 8 years of practice we have 83.96% positive results with one maneuver, 92.68% positive results with 2 maneuvers, recurrence 4.22%.

Some European teams to whom the maneuver has been correctly taught have similar results: R. Boniver (Belgium); J.P. Demanez (Belgium) 90% with 2 maneuvers; G. Guidetti (Italy) 90% within 3 maneuvers; A. Hadj Djilani (Switzerland) 86%; R. Hausler (Switzerland) 84%; J. and C. Robert (France) 95% with 2 maneuvers.

Discussion

The maneuver obviously works. The results are reproducible in other hands than the authors' and are of scientific value. The results have nothing to do with the average time of spontaneous disappearance of the attacks. Some patients had suffered from BPPV for 20–30 years and were cured with one maneuver.

The results have nothing to do with habituation either, because when the maneuver is carried out on normals nothing can be seen or recorded. The results confirm the hypothesis of the cupula being modified in its density, but cannot discriminate between cupulolithiasis and floating substances.

The fact that patients not suffering from vertigo (10% of idiopathic cases of BPPV) sometimes complain of a 'floating sensation' when lying on the side — manifested by a small downward nystagmus that persists and does not revert with orthostatism — might suggest another hypothesis for the etiology of BVVP: i.e. biomechanical dysfunction of the cupula due to variations of pressure between perilymph and endolymph.

References

1   Dix, M.R.; Hallpike, C.S.: The pathology, symptomatology and diagnosis of certain common disorders of the vestibular system. Proc. R. Soc. Med. *45:* 341–354 (1952).
2   Katsarkas, A.; Outerbridge, J.S.: Nystagmus of paroxysmal positional vertigo. Ann. Otol. Rhinol. Lar. *92:* 146–150 (1983).

3   Gacek, R.R.: Further observations on posterior ampullary nerve transsection for positional vertigo. Ann. Otol. Rhinol. Lar. *87:* 300–305 (1978).
4   Norre, E.; Dveerd, W.: Principes et élaboration d'une technique de rééducation vestibulaire: le vestibular habituation training. Annls oto-lar. *96:* 217–227 (1979).
5   Schuknecht, H.F.: Pathology of the ear, pp. 465–473 (Harvard University Press, Cambridge 1974).
6   Stahle, J.; Terrins, J.: Paroxysmal positional nystagmus. Ann. Otol. Rhinol. Lar. *74:* 69–83 (1965).
7   Baloh, R.W.; Sakala, S.M.; Honrubia, V.: Benign paroxysmal positional vertigo. Am. J. Otolaryngol. *1:* 1–6 (1979).
8   Semont, A.; Sterkers, J.M.: Rééducation vestibulaire. Cah. ORL *15:* 305 309 (1980).
9   Semont, A.: Le traitement du VPPB. Traitement des troubles vestibulo-oculaires. Prix médical pour l'amélioration de la qualité de la vie (Bibliothèque de l'Académie Nationale de Médecine, Paris 1984).
10 Cannoni, C.: Le vertige paroxystique bénin; thèse de doctorat en médecine, Marseille (1986).

A. Semont, MD, Vestibular Rehabilitation, 29, rue de la Santé,
F–75013 Paris (France)

Adv. Oto-Rhino-Laryng., vol. 42, pp. 294–300 (Karger, Basel 1988)

Computation of Eye-Head Movements in Oscillopsic Patients: Modifications Induced by Reeducation[1]

G. Freyss, E. Vitte, A. Semont, P. Tran ba Huy, P. Gaillard

ORL Department, Hôpital Lariboisière, Paris, France

One of the most common complaints in daily ENT practice is dizziness caused by head turning. Only one third of our patients suffering from bilateral loss of vestibular function complain of long-standing oscillopsias. Here again, we did not find correlations between standard test — caloric, vestibulo-ocular reflex (VOR), pursuit and saccadic eye movements — and symptoms. Normally eye-head movements are induced by the visual appearance of an interesting lateral target. The patient's eye makes a saccade to catch the target, then a compensatory eye movement is made to stabilize the gaze (hold) (standard paradigm).

Many authors [11, 13] have studied these types of movements in patients with bilateral loss of labyrinthine function. This paradigm is made up of two sequences: an acquisition saccade, then a compensatory eye movement. The interaction between these two movements is important and depends on the relative eye-head movement's timing [12]. We have been studying this paradigm for 4 years in clinical practice. The interpretation is very complex. This is the reason why we chose to study only the compensatory eye movement induced by head movements while the patient tries to stabilize his gaze.

Patients and Methods

Fourteen patients have a complete absence of caloric responses on both sides to standard bithermal stimulation. The diagnoses in the bilateral group were: bilateral

[1] Grant: INSERM–226 C.

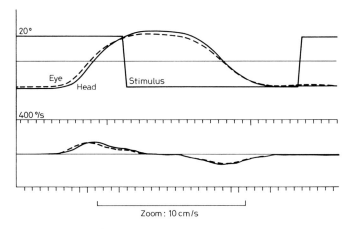

Fig. 1. Normal patient. Eyes opened but covered — the patient is asked to fixate on his extended thumb (imaginary target, EHIm). Top trace = head movements (20°); interrupted line = eye movements (inverted electrodes); bottom trace = velocities (gain 1).

VIIIth section (acoustic neuroma, 1); aminoglycoside ototoxicity, 12; idiopathic, 1. All patients complained of gait unsteadiness, and 9 of oscillopsia at the time of the first testing.

The second test was done after 3 or 6 months of reeducation. We included also 3 unilateral sections of the VIIIth nerve for untreatable Ménière's disease and 10 normal subjects were used for comparison.

Methods

Eye movements were recorded by EOG, head movements by an optoelectronic device (Hamamatsu). Position and velocity signals were digitally processed on-line by a mini-computer (IN 110) [6] (fig. 1).

Passive and active pseudo-random constant amplitude (40°) head saccades (maximum velocity 216 °/s, SD 17) were produced using paradigms: (1) eyes opened — the patient is fixating on a central real earth-fixed target (EHRe); (2) eyes opened but covered, the subject is asked to fixate on his extended thumb. This produces an imaginary target (EHIm).

Data were compared with: (1) cervico-ocular reflex (COR); (2) VOR — rotating chair in pseudo-random saccades with head fixed to a chair using the two same paradigms (central real earth-fixed target or eyes opened but covered fixating on the same remembered target). Results were expressed as gain (mean peak) eye velocity/(mean peak) head velocity.

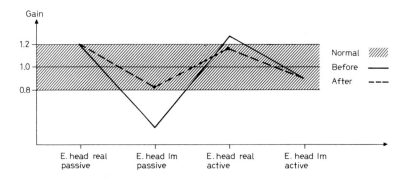

Fig. 2. Gain (mean peak eye velocity/mean peak head velocity) variations in gentamycin areflexic patients, before and after reeducation, compared to the normal range.

Results

Maximum velocity for free head movements wass 209°/s, SD 48°. Maximum chair velocity was 123 °/s, SD 10°. In normal subjects the gain for passive EHRe was 1, SD 0.15, for passive EHIm 0.93, SD 0.10, for active EHRe 0.94, SD 0.06; for active EHIm 0.88, SD 0.12; for VVOR 0.95, SD 0.06, and finally for VOR 0.94, SD 0.15 (fig. 2).

The maximum velocities of the patient's head movements were lower than those of the ENT department's assistants. COR measurements with Thoden's [10] technique gave us low and no reproducible results with our patients. So we used to appreciate the COR by comparison between free head movements and VOR.

Results in normal patients and in patients with bilateral caloric areflexia (gentamycin or idiopathic) are shown in figure 2 before and after reeducation. We notice two points: (1) the gain of passive EHIm is low before reeducation and quite normal after; (2) the gain of the VOR is quite similar to EHIm gain.

The patient with bilateral neurectomy has a gain of 1.29 with real target and VVOR, while with imaginary target and VOR, gain was zero (fig. 3). Active head movements induced anticompensatory eye movements but this test was difficult to perform for this totally deaf female patient.

A number of patients with symptoms before reeducation, especially patients with unilateral vestibular section, cannot carry out active EHIm. Their recordings were similar to recordings with standard paradigm (as if the

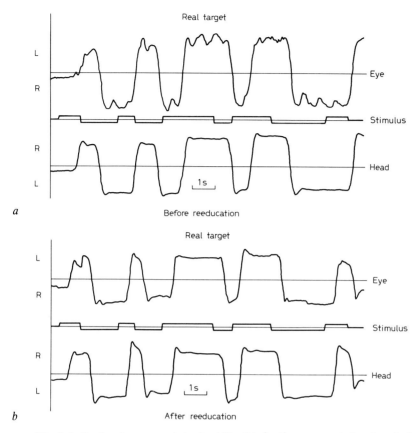

Fig. 3. Active head movements (patient No. 5 is fixating on a central real earth-fixed target). *a* Before reeducation — notice the eye oscillations induced by brisk head movements. *b* After reeducation — normal compensatory eye movements.

patients looked at 2 lateral imaginary targets). This group of patients showed an asymmetric gain with real targets while gain was near zero for VOR in acute stages (these patients stayed for about 7 days in bed). Good improvement was seen after reeducation (fig. 4).

Discussion

Practically all the patients with bilateral caloric areflexia are able, in a few days, to stabilize their gaze on a real target. These compensatory

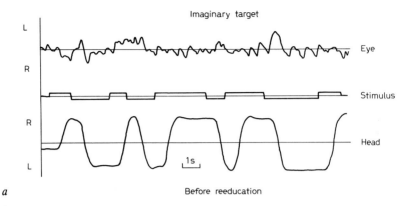

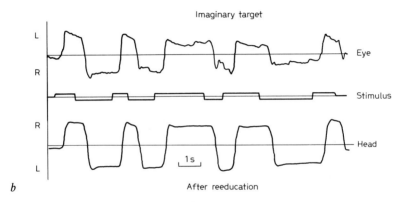

Fig. 4. Passive head movements — imaginary target. Patient No. 10 = unilateral neurectomy. *a* 7th day after unilateral section, there is no compensatory eye movement induced by head turning. *b* After 8 days of reeducation, the gain is quite normal (notice the spontaneous nystagmus).

movements came from the visual system. Before reeducation, some of them made large compensatory saccades that have all the characteristics of visual saccades (eye maximum velocities higher than those of the head).

After reeducation, quite all the patients are making movements of large amplitudes copied exactly on head movements. Maximum velocities are higher than those of the pursuit system and lower than those of visual saccades. Eye velocity curves are similar to vestibular movements and formed of small saccades (overlapping saccades) [9]. So the saccadic system

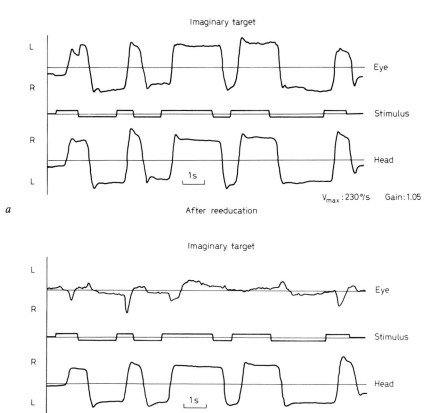

Fig. 5. Passive eye-head movements (imaginary target) without visual feedback after reeducation. Notice the reappearance of normal compensatory eye movements in the gentamycin areflexic patient (a) and their lack in the patient with bilateral neurectomy (b).

is supplying failures of the vestibular system. (It is the same when there is a problem with the pursuit system.)

Before reeducation, patients with gentamycin-induced areflexia produce compensatory movements without vision. Their velocities are not homogeneous (several peaks). The mean of maximum velocities is lower than those of the head. After several months of reeducation, velocities are quite similar. Berthoz [2] has been studying a similar group of patients with an 'off axis rotation technique' (B. Cohen, Barany Society). In this group, they showed that otolithic function is quite normal despite lack of semicircular function (fig. 5).

This result strongly supports our hypothesis that appearance of a normal eye-head coordination in the absence of any visual cue is produced through otolithic input in this group of patients. Again we did not observe such a normalization of eye-head coordination without vision in the patient with bilateral neurectomy.

References

1   Baloh, R.V.; Hess, K.; Honrubia, V.; Yee, R.D.: Low and high frequency sinusoidal rotational testing in patients with peripheral vestibular lesions. Acta oto-lar. suppl. 406, pp. 189–193 (1984).

2   Berthoz, A.: Adaptive mechanisms in eye head coordination; in Berthoz, Melvill-Jones, Adaptive mechanisms in gaze control, pp. 177–202 (Elsevier, Amsterdam 1985).

3   Denise, P.; Corvisier, J.; Vidal, P.P.; Berthoz, A.: Active recentering role of orienting horizontal eye-head synergy after labyrinthine lesions; in Zee, Keller, Adaptive process in visual and oculomotor systems (Pergamon Press, Oxford 1986).

4   Denise, P.: Rotation d'axe incliné par rapport à la gravité, essai des petits angles. Intérêts cliniques; thèse, Paris (1986).

5   Dichgans, J.; Bizzi, E.; Morasso, D.: The role of vestibular and neck afferents during eye-head coordination in the monkey. Brain Res. *71:* 225–232 (1974).

6   Freyss, G.; Vitte, E.; Pialoux, P.: Nystagmographie. Encyclopéd. Méd. Chir. ORL 20199 M10 (1984).

7   Melvill-Jones, G.: Adaptive behavior; in Berthoz, Melvill-Jones, Adaptive mechanisms in gaze control, p. 196 (Elsevier, Amsterdam 1985).

8   Pulaski, D.; Zee, D.; Robinson, D.A.: The behavior of the vestibulo-ocular reflex at high velocities of head rotation. Brain Res. *222:* 159–165 (1981).

9   Stark, L.: Eye-head coordination: neurological control of active gaze. Proc. 2[e] Congr. Aerospatial, Toulouse 1983, pp. 63–73.

10   Thoden, U.; Doerr, M.; Leopold, C.: Motion perception of head or trunk modulates cervico-ocular reflex (COR). Acta oto-lar. *96:* 9–14 (1983).

11   Takahashi, M.; Uemurat, T.; Fujishiro, T.: Compensatory eye movement and gaze fixation during active head rotation in patients with labyrinthine disorders. Ann. Otol. Rhinol. Lar. *90:* 241–245 (1981).

12   Zangemeister, W.; Stark, L.: Gaze latency: variable interactions of head and eye latency. Expl Neurol. *77:* 563–577 (1982).

13   Zee, D.; Eye-head coordination; in Leigh, Zee, The neurology of eye movement, pp. 109–124 (Davis, Philadelphia 1983).

G. Freyss, MD, ORL Department, Hôpital Lariboisière, 2 Rue Ambroise Paré, F–75010 Paris (France)

Subject Index